Preface	i
1. Who is this book for?	1
2. What is Meridian Systems Yoga	2
3. Acupuncture	3
4. Principles of TCM	4
5. Yin & Yang	6
6. The Five Fundamental Substances	8
Jing	8
Qi	9
Shen	10
Blood	11
Fluids	11
7. Meridians	12
8. Organs & Meridians	14
Lung and Large Intestine	16
Spleen and Stomach	20
Heart and Small Intestine	23
Kidney and Urinary Bladder	25
Pericardium and Triple Burner	29
Liver and Gallbladder	32
The Governing and Conception Vessels	35
9. Meridian groups	39

10. Designing your practice	40
Vary Your Practice	40
Length of Holding the Poses	41
Breath	41
Length of practice	42
Day, Time and Frequency of Practice	42
Location of Your Practice	43
MERIDIAN SYSTEMS YOGA ASANAS	45
11. Meridian Systems Yoga Asanas	46
Anterior Thorax	48
Lateral Thorax	54
Posterior Thorax	64
Three Arm Yin and Three Arm Yang	68
Three Leg Yin and Three Leg Yang	76
MERIDIAN SYSTEMS YOGA ASANA SEQUENCES	83
12. Meridian Systems Yoga Asana Sequences	84
Anterior & Lateral Thorax, Three Leg Yin & Three Leg Yang	84
Anterior & Posterior Thorax, Three Leg Yin & Three Leg Yang #1	87
Anterior & Posterior Thorax, Three Leg Yin & Three Leg Yang #2	89
Three Arm Yin & Three Arm Yang	91
All Meridian Groups Asana Sequence	93
Bibliography	95

Meridian Systems
YOGA

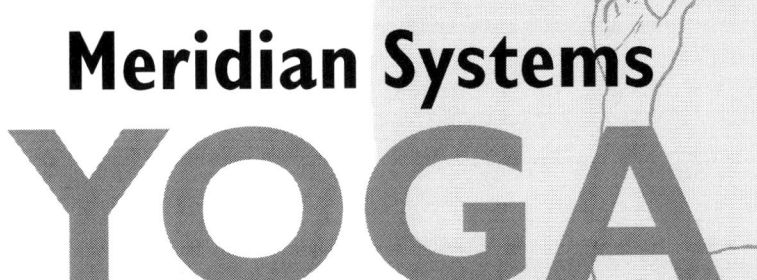

**An Accessible & Innovative Method
Combining Yoga & Traditional Chinese Medicine**

*A Method for People of All Ages,
Body Types, & Fitness Levels*

LEE L. HERRERA

MSY Publications • Santa Fe, NM

Meridian Systems Yoga
Published by MSY Publications 2015
Santa Fe, New Mexico

© Lee L. Herrera, 2015.

All rights reserved. No part of this book may be reproduced, stored in a retrieval system, or transmitted, in any form or by any means, electronic, mechanical, photocopying, recording, or otherwise, without the written permission of the author.

Printed in the United States of America by CreateSpace

Cover and interior design by Ann Lowe

Models:
    Ann Mauzy
    Deedee Jansen
    Lee Herrera
    Robert Bookwalter

Illustrations by Samara Reigh

ISBN 978-1514126011

PREFACE

THIS BOOK IS THE OUTCOME of twenty years of personal yoga practice and of receiving acupuncture treatments. In the summer of 2007, I decided to try acupuncture for the first time. A new alternative medicine clinic opened up a few blocks away from my apartment at the time in Seattle. The clinic director, Teri Adolfo, stood outside and handed out flyers with the clinic's various services. I was curious and called the next day to schedule an appointment. I arrived straight after work, tired and a feeling a little stressed. I knew nothing about acupuncture or Chinese medicine and didn't know what to expect. Teri took my pulses after I lay down on the treatment table. She then took out a box of acupuncture needles and inserted them in specific points on my body. Almost instantly I started feeling a very pleasant flow of energy. I later learned that it was Qi that was being stimulated within my meridians. After forty-five minutes of treatment both the tiredness and the stress completely went away. Instead, I felt relaxed and peaceful. I was very fascinated by the treatment, so I scheduled another one for the following week. The dramatic change in my overall emotional well-being repeated itself once again, and I began receiving two acupuncture treatments per month. I also started wondering how acupuncture actually worked. I remember asking myself how a few little needles stuck in my upper arm could alter the way I felt. I also wondered if maybe yoga asanas (postures) that stimulate the same anatomical region could bring forth a similar affect.

In the next few months, I read a couple of introductory acupuncture and Chinese Medicine books and I bought meridian charts. I then started to design a yoga practice according to the location of the meridians in my body. Teri diagnosed me with Kidney Qi deficiency and Lung Qi deficiency. I therefore practiced yoga asanas that stimulated the anatomical regions where those meridians are located (three arm yin, anterior thorax, & three leg yin meridian groups). To my amazement, both the physical and emotional symptoms related to those meridians began to improve. I was more energized and I didn't stress so much at work. Instead, I was much more accepting and was able to remain calm and happy throughout the day.

In the following months I made another important discovery. I realized that basic yoga asanas stimulate Qi and remove Qi blockages within the meridians just as well as the very complex ones. Most of the asanas in this book are variations of existing yoga asanas. I made them simple so they could easily fit the needs of anyone. I soon figured that I could develop a yoga method that would be accessible to anyone who wished to enjoy the benefits of yoga, regardless of their body type, age, or fitness level.

Creating a yoga method that was totally accessible was especially important and meaningful for me. Over the years I've heard many people complain that they could not do yoga because they were intimidated by it. "I can't compete with all the other young and super flexible students in class" was a common response. Others felt that they were just too old, too stiff, or just not good enough. I personally believe that yoga is a healing modality that ought to be accessible to anyone, not just a limited population of young, slender, and fit people. I also believe that the basic principles and applications of Traditional Chinese Medicine should be more widely available. Both modalities hold vast knowledge and wisdom and have an amazing potential to help people improve their overall health and well-being. They should therefore be available for everyone to practice. The goal of Meridian Systems Yoga is just that: to make yoga and Traditional Chinese Medicine accessible to everyone. It works for me, it works for many of my students, and I hope it'll work for you too.

CHAPTER

Who is this book for?

THIS BOOK IS FOR ANYONE who wishes to improve his or her physical and emotional well-being through yoga in a simple and accessible practice. Meridian Systems Yoga is designed for people of all ages, body types, and fitness levels - from people that have never before practiced yoga to lifetime yogis. It is an interdisciplinary method that allows people to achieve physical and emotional well-being by utilizing simple elements of traditional yoga combined with Traditional Chinese Medicine (TCM). By using simple yoga asanas (poses), Meridian Systems Yoga turns both yoga and TCM into a simple, accessible, and universal practice that can easily fit the needs and ability levels of anyone. It is not necessary to be fit and flexible in order to incorporate more well-being, love, and happiness and into your life.

CHAPTER 2

What is Meridian Systems Yoga?

MERIDIAN SYSTEMS YOGA uses yoga asanas to stimulate Qi flow and remove Qi blockages of particular meridian groups in the body. In Traditional Chinese Medicine (TCM), emotions are an intrinsic aspect of meridians (which will be explained at more length later in the book), thus this is a system that achieves holistic balance at the physical, emotional, and spiritual levels. This method works similarly to acupuncture and provides the means to focus one's practice on specific physical and emotional concerns.

CHAPTER 3

Acupuncture

ACUPUNCTURE WORKS TO achieve a balance between Yin and Yang and to harmonize the various organs and energies of the body. Meridian Systems Yoga also focuses on meridian balance and harmony, but with yoga asanas instead of acupuncture needles. Meridian Systems Yoga utilizes the meridians of TCM and their emotional correspondences, providing a simplification of both yoga and TCM and a deepening of their basic principles.

CHAPTER 4

Principles of TCM

THIS BOOK, AND TCM LITERATURE in general, often refer to the organs and meridians in singular form (e.g. the Lung meridian, Kidney Qi etc.). It is important to note that the meridians run through both sides of the body symmetrically. The meridian diagrams too illustrate the meridians as if they ran through one side of the body only. In reality, they run through both sides, as a mirror image.

A basic understanding of Traditional Chinese Medicine is necessary to understand Meridian Systems Yoga. TCM is rooted in ancient traditions and philosophies, and focuses on the individual in metaphorical terms rather than purely anatomical terms. Its system of medicine understands health via the functionality and interrelation of all the various parts of the body. When there is disharmony in the activity of the whole, emotional imbalance and ill health will arise. This interconnectedness is a defining aspect of TCM. Western medicine usually identifies pathologies with only one disease process or body part as the object of examination, and then utilizes pharmacological or surgical treatments to address this specifically. TCM, on the other hand, identifies patterns of disharmony, and uses acupuncture and herbs to bring the elements of the body, emotions, and spirit back into a state of health and harmony. This is not to disparage the wonderful and impressive aspects of Western Medicine, but merely to emphasize the differences between these two medical traditions, and to emphasis TCM's holistic perception of the body.

For the purpose of illustrating the theory of Meridian System Yoga, this book will address only a few concepts of TCM: Yin and Yang, Jing, Qi, Shen, Blood, Fluids, Meridians, and Organs.

CHAPTER 5

Yin & Yang

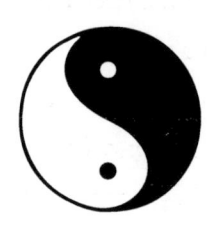

YIN AND YANG are the concepts that comprise the foundation of the Chinese medical theory. They are understood as the two complementary parts of the One. Yin and Yang are used to describe how things function in relation to one another, and they illustrate how change and relationship occur. For example:

YIN	YANG
Night	Day
Inactivity	Activity
Rest	Motion
Fall & Winter	Spring & Summer
Cold	Hot
Water	Fire
Shaded	Sunny
Front of the Body	Back of the Body
Inside of the Body	Outside of the Body

While certain things are called 'Yin' and other things 'Yang,' in reality, the two cannot be separated. Yin makes Yang possible, and Yang makes Yin possible. For example, the energetic, active motion of the body

(Yang) is nourished and made possible by times of restful inactivity (Yin). The Taoist yin-yang symbol expresses the principle of these merging opposites: in the black of Yin is the small seed of Yang; in the white of Yang is the small seed of yin. Yin and Yang *create* and *transform* one another. In late winter, we see the first signs of spring – birds returning, new plants pushing up through the soil, a warm-smelling breeze. In late summer, we see the hints of coming autumn – birds departing, leaves browning, the sweet scent of rot. Just so, Yin transforms into Yang and Yang transforms into Yin.

Yin and Yang also *balance* one another and cannot exist without the other, an important aspect in health. When Yin and Yang fall into disharmony, we see illness. When Yin is deficient and not controlling Yang (or if Yang is excessive and overpowering Yin), a person may be feverish, angry, and red-faced. In Western terms, this could manifest in many different forms, such as hypertension, stroke, or migraines. In TCM, it is understood as too much fire (Yang) evaporating the body's cooling and relaxing water (Yin). When Yang is deficient and not controlling Yin (or if Yin is excessive and overpowering Yang), the individual could be cold, lethargic, and pale. This could manifest as hypothyroidism, depression, or chronic fatigue syndrome. Too much water drenches the body's energetic and metabolic fire.

Everything we experience is part of the dynamic interrelation of Yin and Yang.

CHAPTER 6

The Five Fundamental Substances

THE FIVE FUNDAMENTAL SUBSTANCES are Jing, Qi, Shen, Blood and Fluids. We will describe the principles of Jing, Qi and Shen in more depth but their interrelation can be understood as the three basic vibrational frequencies of the body. *Jing* is the roots of a tree, reaching deep into the earth, deriving underground sustenance, and keeping the body stable and grounded. *Qi* is the trunk of the tree, active and growing, keeping the balance between the downward motion of the roots and the upward motion of the branches. *Shen* is the branches, leaves and fruit of the tree, reaching toward the heavens, a higher consciousness and understanding of the self as a part of a greater whole.

JING

Jing is referred to as "essence," a rarified substance that carries us from conception to death. It is largely derived from our parents (pre-natal Jing) and often referred to as our genetic makeup, our roots. Jing governs reproduction and development. Birth defects, delayed puberty, infertility, premature aging, or developmental delays are often interpreted as deficient Jing. Jing is also acquired during our lives, though in smaller amounts, as the purified parts of food and water. While it is easy to deplete Jing through stress, an imbalanced lifestyle, and exhausted adrenals, it is very difficult to replenish it. Thus, Jing is understood as something to be preserved and cherished. Jing is stored and replenished by the Kidneys.

QI

Qi is similar to the idea of *prana* in the yogic tradition. *Qi* has often been translated as "energy," but the most important aspect of Qi is not what it *is*, but rather what it *does*. Qi is Yang in nature, and thus is concerned with motion, activity, and functionality. It exists in the world around us and within our bodies. Qi has been described in many different ways—as electricity running through our body, as rivers of energy, or as our basic vital force—regardless of the metaphor, Qi is always in motion. When Qi is blocked, we may feel frustrated or stagnant.

Both yoga and Chinese Medicine work to unblock Qi and keep the energy of the body flowing harmoniously. Yoga uses asanas and breathing to keep the body oxygenated and flexible, thus facilitating the movement of Qi. Acupuncture identifies specific locations of Qi blockage and uses specific points on meridians to release the stagnant Qi. Similar to acupuncture, Meridian Systems Yoga uses a unique set of asanas and asana sequences to harmonize the functions of the meridians.

While Qi has many important and varied functions, we will focus on Meridian Qi—the Qi that flows through the meridians of the body and harmonizes the activity of the organs into a working whole. Imbalances in the Meridian Qi creates patterns of emotional and physical disease.

The two major sources of Qi imbalance are a deficiency of Qi or a blockage of Qi. Consider a river that flows to a lake, filling it with fresh water. The river is a meridian and the lake is an organ. If the river has debris obstructing its flow, it cannot fill the lake with pure water. The result will be ill health. Qi blockages may manifest themselves physically or emotionally. Physically, Qi blockages may be observed as pain; headaches, stomachaches, pain in the rib cage, muscular tension (especially in the back and shoulders), or pain along the meridians. Emotionally, Qi blockages may be observed as stagnant emotions or the feeling of being "stuck" with such emotions as stress, irritability, anxiety, anger, frustration, sadness, grief, and depression.

Insufficient water in the river is another situation in which the lake (the organ) will not receive pure water (Qi). This could be due to drought (poor diet and dehydration), the spring running dry (physiological disturbances, illness), or the river being diverted for other purposes (stress, overwork, excessive activity). The name in TCM for the river providing insufficient water to the lake is *deficient Qi*. TCM pairs this with another important concept, *deficient Blood*, but as the health of Blood is treated primarily through diet and herbs, we will be focusing on Qi.

SHEN

Shen is understood as "spirit." It is the consciousness, ideas, and vibrancy of the individual. The state of Shen can often be observed in the eyes. A healthy Shen will be present and lively, conscious of the surroundings and of self. An unhealthy Shen may be seen in muddled or shifty eyes that do not seem to accurately evaluate situations; in extreme forms, a Shen disharmony may be interpreted as mental illness.

While Shen is often translated as "mind," it is important to distinguish between the Chinese and Western conceptions of mind. In the Western world, mind is equated with "brain." In the TCM understanding, mind is Shen: the collective workings of the consciousness, the spirit, and the heart-center.

BLOOD

TCM's Blood is similar to, but not the same as, the Western conception of "blood." In TCM, Blood is conceptualized as the nourishing force that runs through the body. Qi is the active Yang force that circulates the body, bringing energy to all its moving parts, and Blood is its Yin counterpart, regulating and moistening the internal pathways and organs. Like Qi, Blood may be deficient or stagnant.

FLUIDS

Fluids are all the bodily fluids apart from Blood. Together they moisten the skin, hair, joints, muscles, bones, organs, brain, spinal cord and membranes of the body. Fluids include saliva, sweat, tears, gastric fluid, and urine. They are considered Yin substances, as their nature is like water.

CHAPTER 7

Meridians

MERIDIANS are also called "channels" in TCM, and may be imagined as the streams and rivers of the body through which Qi and Blood flow. Just as a river may be blocked by debris or a dam, so too can meridians become obstructed. As will be explained in the coming chapters, Meridian Systems Yoga utilizes yoga asanas to stimulate Qi flow and release Qi blockages within the meridians.

Another way to understand meridians is to imagine them as electrical circuits that run through the body, bringing Qi to all the parts, linking the organs in a single dynamic system. According to TCM, when this flow of Qi is obstructed or imbalanced, illness arises. Furthermore, a disharmony in an organ may appear as discomfort in its corresponding meridian. For example, obstruction in the Heart can manifest as pain radiating down the medial aspect of the arm, all the way to the palm—the course of the Heart meridian.

In Chinese Medicine, meridians are associated with specific internal organs, which in turn govern specific emotions. Thus, through stimulating meridian Qi flow and unblocking its flow through Meridian Systems

Yoga asanas, we can affect our emotional well-being. Imagine a branch of a tree with an apple growing at its tip. The branch is the meridian and the apple is the organ. Disorders within the meridians lead to disorders within the organs, and disorders within the organs lead to emotional imbalances. Conversely, imbalanced emotions over a long period of time may lead to organ dysfunction, meridian pain or Qi blockage, and eventually illness.

Meridians connect the inside of the body to the outside of the body, Yin to Yang, and the organs to one another. They are the framework of our physical and energetic body. The meridian system unifies all the different parts and functions of the body.

CHAPTER 8

Organs and Meridians

IN BOTH WESTERN MEDICINE AND TCM, physical and emotional health is interrelated. Physical health affects emotional well-being, just as our emotional state affects physical health. For example, if someone is in chronic excruciating pain, his or her emotions are likely to suffer as well. Or, if someone has a career and home life with constant stress, he or she will probably see corresponding health pathologies, like high blood pressure or adrenal fatigue.

Whereas Western medicine understand the organs foremost as physical structures, and bases its analysis on quantifiable substances, TCM focuses on the functionality of organs and seeks to regulate their activities into a more harmonious whole. In TCM, emotions are understood as energetic qualities that result from and contribute to the functions of the organs. Proper functioning of the organs sustains harmony on physical, mental, and spiritual planes. Harmony is achieved when the organs, Jing, Qi, Shen, Blood, and body fluids all work together as a dynamic whole. The goal of Meridian Systems Yoga is to achieve this harmony.

The twelve organs in Chinese Medicine and their corresponding meridians are as follows:

Lung	Kidney
Large Intestine	Urinary Bladder
Spleen	Pericardium
Stomach	Triple Burner
Heart	Liver
Small Intestine	Gallbladder

The organs are divided into two groups: Yin and Yang organs. The Yin organs create, transform, store, and manage the Jing, Qi, Shen, Blood and Fluids of the body, whereas the Yang organs take a more active role in transporting, breaking down, absorbing, and excreting Qi, Blood, Fluids, food, and waste. Each Yin organ has a Yang counterpart; together they are called Yin-Yang partner organs.

The partnered organs are:
  Lungs (Yin) and Large Intestine (Yang)   *Autumn*
  Spleen (Yin) and Stomach (Yang)
  Heart (Yin) and Small Intestine (Yang)
  Kidney (Yin) and Urinary Bladder (Yang)
  Pericardium (Yin) and Triple Burner (Yang)
  Liver (Yin) and Gallbladder (Yang)

The emotions associated with these Yin-Yang pairs tend to focus on the Yin aspect, but the Yang manifestations are also important. We will briefly address the emotional and physiological functions of these pairs—there is a wealth of information on the nature of these organs, but for the purposes of this book, we will focus on a simple understanding of the concepts. A supplemental reading list on both yoga and TCM can be found at the end the book. The organ system of TCM is very detailed and complex, encompassing many nuances and pathologies that we do not have space to describe, and is not necessary for an understanding of Meridian Systems Yoga. For the purposes of this book, simple conceptions of the organs and their associated emotions are used to select appropriate asanas and asana sequences.

While TCM identifies a large number of patterns of disharmony—within the Liver organ & meridian system alone, we can see Liver Blood Deficiency, Liver Blood Stasis, Excess Liver Yang, Liver Fire Blazing, Liver Yin Deficiency, Liver Qi Stagnation, Rebellious Liver Qi, Rebellious Liver Qi Invading the Spleen, Damp-Heat in the Liver-Gallbladder channels . . . the list goes on. These different patterns have different symptoms. For the purposes of this book, we will merely identify what it looks like when the Liver is in harmony and when it is in disharmony. Students who wish to more deeply understand the diagnostic patterns of TCM may refer to the list of additional reading materials.

LUNG AND LARGE INTESTINE

Lung

The Lungs govern the breath of the body. This process occurs on many levels. On a physical level, we know that the lungs are responsible for respiration. On an energetic level, the Lungs derive Qi from the air, extracting the "pure" aspect for circulation and oxygenation of the body, and exhaling the "impure" aspects. Lungs are said to "govern the Qi of the body."

Organs and Meridians   17

The health of the Lungs is what protects us from external pathogens and diseases. The Lungs control our "defensive Qi," which is our immune system. If someone has a poor immune system and is always catching colds, he or she likely has a Lung deficiency. The Lungs also control the skin, and thus issues like eczema or psoriasis may be attributed to a disharmony of the Lungs. Physical dysfunction of the Lungs may also manifest as asthma and chronic cough.

The Lungs lets us breathe in what is good and to exhale what is no longer needed. A Lung disharmony manifests in several ways emotionally, but all are related to the basic function of inhaling and exhaling freely. We will focus on two of these ways. One way is when a person tries too hard to hold on to loved ones, a place, a job, a way of thinking or acting, and thus is unwilling to exhale and let things progress naturally. Such a person might be called "uptight" or "a perfectionist." The Lungs has the duty of taking in inspiration (an idea, a revelation—something that is *inspired* or *breathed in*) and transforming it into reality, *exhaling* its existence into the world. When a person gets stuck on the process of breathing in, and is unwilling to breathe out and accept change, they become rigid in their beliefs.

Another manifestation of Lung disharmony is when a person gets stuck on the exhale. They live in a permanent sigh. This could happen after the loss of a

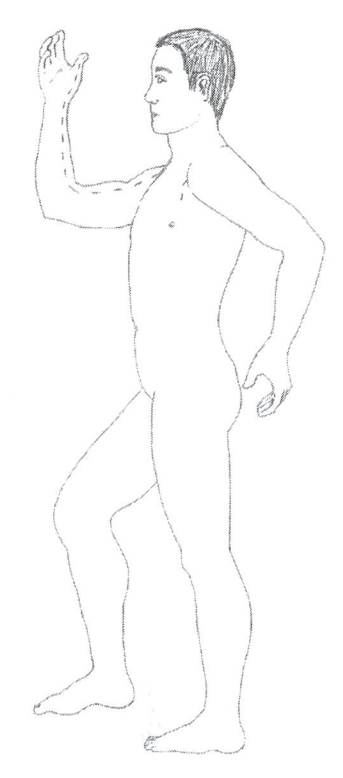

Three Arm Yin Meridian Group (medial)

THE LUNG meridian originates on the lateral aspect of the chest in the first intercostal space. It runs down the arm to the elbow, then to the wrist, ending at the radial border of the thumb's fingernail.

loved one, for example. While a certain amount of grief is necessary and good, a person may become lodged in this state of mourning for longer than is healthy. They could be in a state of depression, seemingly without cause. These individuals are fixated on the sadness of letting go, on the melancholy of the exhale, and are unwilling to inhale and open themselves to the new. (There are other causes of depression, addressed in the Liver chapter).

It is often observed that when people do not wish to address pain or grief, they smoke, damaging the lungs instead of allowing them to process sorrow.

Harmony
- healthy respiration
- strong immune system
- inspired and alert
- can experience grief and subsequently let go of grief when the time comes

Disharmony
- poor immune system
- cough
- bright pale complexion
- dry throat, dry skin, dry mouth, excessive thirst
- shallow or difficult breathing
- shortness of breath
- allergies
- quiet voice & dislike of speaking
- sinus congestion
- long-lasting grief
- melancholy depression
- lack of inspiration / apathy
- despondency

Large Intestine

The Large Intestine absorbs water and excretes waste. Disharmonies in the Large Intestine clinically show themselves as abdominal pain, diarrhea, or constipation. Emotionally, the Large Intestine can be seen as our ability to "let go" of things. The Lungs and Large Intestine are partner organs and thus intertwined in their emotional associations – grief is closely tied to our ability to let go.

In their harmonious aspect, we can see the Lungs receiving inspiration, putting it to use in an idea or invention, and the Large Intestine sharing it with others. The Large Intestine is known as "The Disseminator of the Tao." While we generally think of the Large Intestine as merely releasing waste into the world, we can also interpret it metaphorically as releasing what we have *processed and understood* into the world, sharing what we have learned.

Harmony
    regular, formed stools
    ability to effectively process and release emotions

Disharmony
    constipation
    hard or dry bowel movements
    blood or mucus in stools
    chronic loose bowel movements
    "holding on to things"

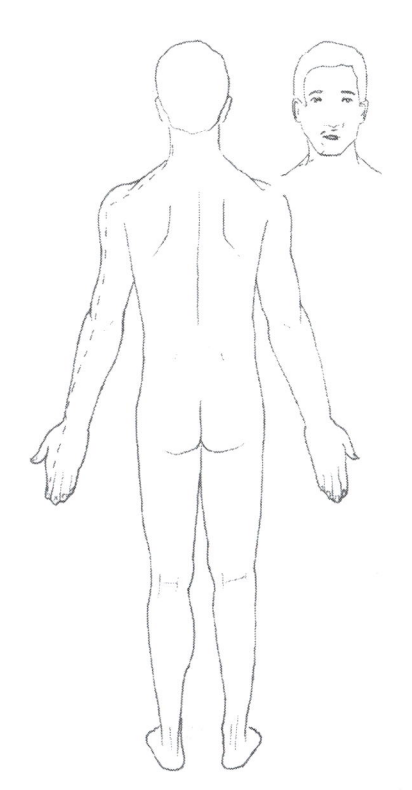

Three Arm Yang Meridian Group (lateral)

THE LARGE INTESTINE meridian begins beside the index finger's nail. It runs up the index finger, up the radial side of the wrist, to the elbow and then the shoulder. It continues up the lateral side of the neck, then crosses the face to the point directly beneath the nostril. It ends lateral to the nose.

Lung & Large Intestine Meridian Groups Asanas
Acceptance

For opening up to new experience, releasing stress, letting go, moving through grief or depression, and for people with respiratory disease or discomfort.
Accepting life as it is.

SPLEEN AND STOMACH

Spleen

The Spleen is in charge of *transforming* and *transporting* food and fluids into Qi and Blood. In TCM, it is understood as the primary organ of digestion and thus has a strong emotional correlation with *nourishment*. Disharmonies in the Spleen almost always result in Qi and Blood deficiency because the Spleen has not properly broken down food to be made into Qi and Blood for the body to use, leading to poor digestion and fatigue. Good diet is immensely important for the Spleen. If someone has a Spleen disharmony, they should focus on eating warm, nutritious foods, and doing so at relaxed times—not reading, standing, arguing with others, or at a desk job. It is important that the Spleen have the resources it needs in order to transform our food into Qi and Blood.

Emotionally, a Spleen disharmony may manifest as neediness and a feeling of not being cared for or loved

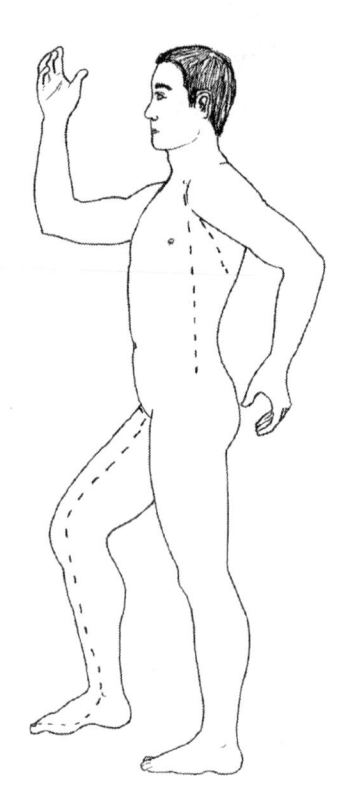

Lateral Thorax Meridian Group
Three Leg Yin Meridian Group (Medial)

THE SPLEEN meridian begins at the medial side of the big toe's nail. It follows the medial aspect of the foot and ascends at the heel to run along the tibia. It continues past the knee and thigh to the lower abdomen. It rises to the lateral aspect of the chest and then drops back down, where it ends in the seventh intercostal space.

enough by others. The Spleen is associated with *worry*, the sort of obsessive, circular thoughts that repeat endlessly with no resolution. People with Spleen Deficiencies often complain of such bothersome thoughts that keep them awake at night. In harmony, when a person feels nourished by loved ones and their environment, the Spleen manifests as a caring, nurturing, motherly force.

Harmony
- healthy eating habits
- strong digestion
- nourishing relationships with friends and family
- clarity of thought and action

Disharmony
- loose stools
- tiredness/lethargy
- bloating
- weak and cold limbs
- organ prolapse (stomach, uterus, anus, or Urinary Bladder)
- "fuzzy-headedness," lack of focus
- poor appetite
- overindulgence in sweet foods
- "neediness"/"clinginess"
- worry & circular thinking

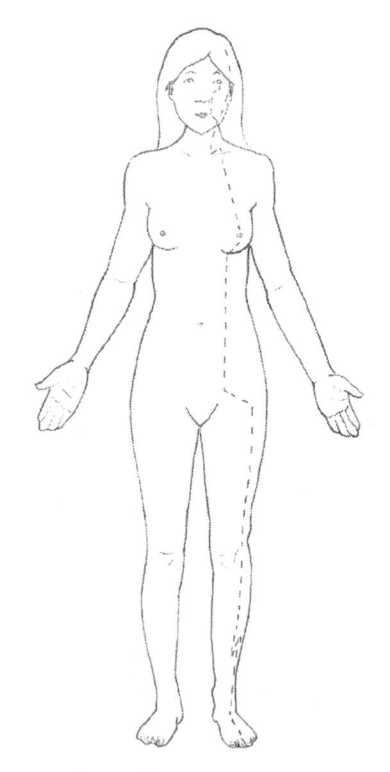

Anterior Thorax Meridian Group
Three Leg Yang Meridian Group (Lateral)

THE STOMACH meridian begins beneath the eye. It descends over the cheek and jaw, then rises to the cheekbone and the lateral aspect of the head. The channel then descends through the neck, clavicle, chest, abdomen, and pelvis. From the hip downward, the Stomach meridian follows the femur and then the lateral side of the tibia. It runs over the top of the ankle and ends on the dorsal aspect of the second toe.

Stomach

The Stomach's duty is to *rot* and *ripen* the food, so that nutrients may be used by the body. It is the counterpart to the Spleen in the process of digestion. The Stomach sends the impure parts of food to the Small Intestine (and then on to the Large Intestine) to be excreted. When the Stomach is in disharmony, we see aggravated digestion. Like the Spleen, many Stomach issues can be addressed through diet—eating nutritious foods at regular times throughout the day.

Emotionally, a person with Stomach disharmony might seem greedy and dissatisfied. They may have an underlying sense that they're "not getting what they need." The Spleen and the Stomach are united in our sense of whether we are being nurtured—both physically and emotionally—by the world around us.

Harmony
    healthy eating habits
    strong digestion
    a feeling of satisfaction and well-being

Disharmony
    stomachache
    nausea
    belching
    acid reflux
    vomiting
    greed & dissatisfaction

Spleen & Stomach Meridian Groups Asanas
Nurture

For feeling nourished by the world, clear thinking, rejuvenating sleep, stronger digestion, better eating habits, and positive relationships with others.

HEART AND SMALL INTESTINE

Heart

The Heart is the home of the Shen, or spirit, and thus is concerned with consciousness, thought, and awareness. The Heart is considered the emperor of the body, regulating and maintaining proper function. The Heart "governs the Blood," and is thus responsible for circulation.

When the Heart is healthy, the individual is in joyful accordance with his or her surroundings—respectful and conscious of his or her place among others. When the Heart is in disharmony, we see insomnia and anxiety, and a variety of mental-emotional disturbances, which may be understood as behavior that is inappropriate for a particular time and place or a distorted understanding of reality.

Harmony
- proper heart functioning
- good sleep
- rational understanding of reality

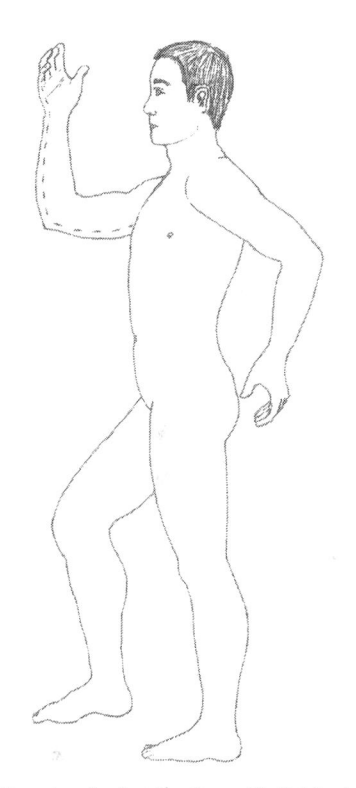

Three Arm Yin Meridian Group (Medial Arm)

THE HEART meridian begins in the center of the armpit. It follows the medial aspect of the arm down the elbow and wrist. It crosses the palm between the fourth and fifth fingers, and ends on the dorsal aspect hand, beside the nail of the little finger.

appropriate behavior
respect for self and others
joy and delight

Disharmony
insomnia
poor blood circulation
feeling the heart beating in the chest
anxiety
inappropriate behavior
manic episodes

Small Intestine

The Small Intestine separates the *pure* from the *turbid*. It receives food from the Stomach and continues the process of decomposition and the absorption of pure aspects of food and fluid. Disharmonies may include abdominal pain, diarrhea, or constipation.

The Small Intestine's emotional duty is to set boundaries; to understand which influences are pure and good, and which are dangerous and unhealthy. The Small Intestine *discriminates*. The Heart and Small Intestine work together to guide us in correct and beneficial interactions with our environment, to have proper boundaries and behave in a way that is respectful of self and of others.

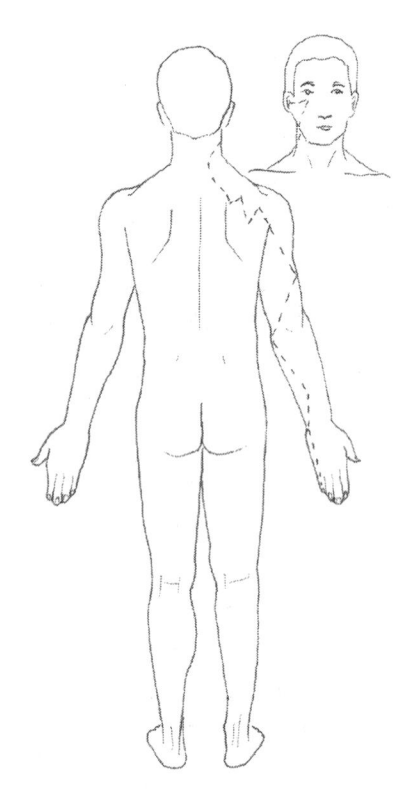

Three Arm Yang Meridian Group (Lateral)

THE SMALL INTESTINE meridian begins on the dorsal aspect of the little finger. It runs past the wrist, up the arm to the elbow and shoulder. It makes a triangle shape on the scapula before crossing up to the neck. On the face, it runs up to the cheek and then ends beside the ear.

Harmony
> healthy digestion
>
> good boundaries

Disharmony
> abdominal pain
>
> digestive disturbances
>
> difficulty setting limits, or tendency to be overly discriminating and strict

Heart & Small Intestine Meridian Groups Asanas
Integrity

For freedom from anxiety, knowing right from wrong, increased intuition, acknowledging proper boundaries, and gaining respect for self and for others. Joyfulness in right action.

KIDNEY AND URINARY BLADDER

Kidney

The Kidneys store Jing, or "essence." They are concerned with growth, development, aging, bones, teeth, ears, and sexual reproduction—the natural and harmonious unfolding of a life from birth to death. Each at its proper time, the fontanel will close on the infant's head, the teeth will come in, the bones will grow longer and stronger, puberty will occur, sexual reproduction will be fruitful, and aging will happen naturally and

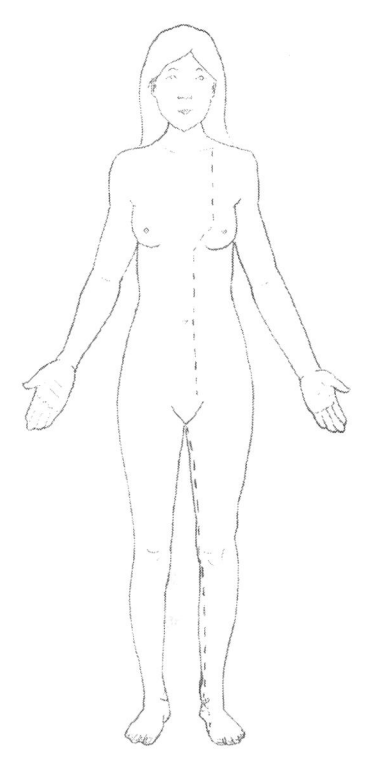

Anterior Thorax Meridian Group
Three Leg Yin Meridian Group (Medial)

THE KIDNEY meridian begins on the sole of the foot. It runs up the side of the foot to the space between the medial malleolus and the Achilles tendon. In line with the Achilles tendon, the Kidney meridian rises up the medial aspect of the leg to the top of the pubic bone. It travels up the lower abdomen, past the umbilicus, up the ribcage, ending beneath the clavicle.

gradually. It is the duty of the Kidneys to make sure that this process goes smoothly. When the Kidneys are out of harmony, clinical manifestations include improper development, sexual dysfunction, as well as metabolic, adrenal, and endocrine disorders.

Kidneys have two aspects: Kidney Yin and Kidney Yang. Kidney Yin stores and circulates Jing. Kidney Yang is the metabolic fire of the body, at the root of all physiological processes. The Yin of the Kidney provides Yin to all the other organs of the body, and the Yang of the Kidney provides Yang. Thus, chronic diseases often are seen in TCM as a Kidney disharmony-when something is wrong on a deep, foundational level, the Kidneys are inevitably involved. Also, chronic poor health, including stress, overwork, and an unbalanced lifestyle without proper rest, end up draining the Kidneys.

Emotionally, the Kidneys are associated with *will*—the reservoir of self-knowledge and destiny that carries us through from birth to death. However, when an individual loses touch with their deep sense of will and self-trust, *fear* dominates instead. Both of these emotions are connected with the Kidney.

Harmony
- healthy bones and growth
- healthy sexual development and activity
- proper hormonal functioning
- normal metabolism
- self-trust
- will power

Disharmony
- impotence (deficient Kidney Yang)
- low libido (deficient Kidney Yang)
- lack of drive or willpower (deficient Kidney Yang)
- chronic fatigue/ feeling "drained" (deficient Kidney Yin and Yang)
- excessive sex drive (deficient Kidney Yin)
- night sweats (deficient Kidney Yin)
- tinnitus (deficient Kidney Yin)
- mental restlessness (deficient Kidney Yin)
- low back pain
- infertility
- improper development (i.e., poor bone development in children, premature graying, delayed puberty)
- poor hearing
- blue-black circles beneath eyes

Urinary Bladder

The duty of the Urinary Bladder is to excrete urine. Disharmonies in the Urinary Bladder include urinary tract infections or incontinence.

Emotionally, the Urinary Bladder manifests *fear*, like its partner organ, the Kidney. The Urinary Bladder displays this as suspiciousness or jealousy. Furthermore, blocked emotions often manifest on the Urinary Bladder meridian as back pain, as this is the primary meridian of the back of the body. Our backs are strong, muscular parts of our body, and thus are often used

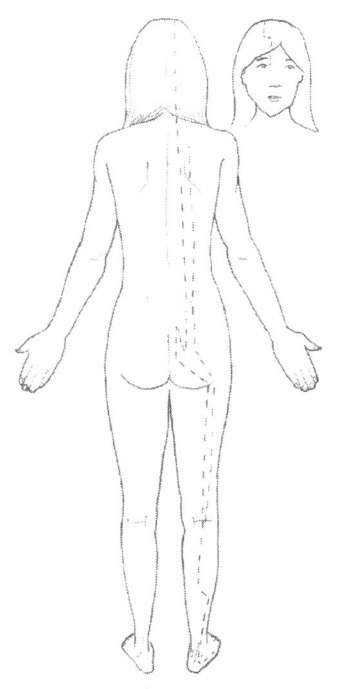

Posterior Thorax Meridian Group
Three Leg Yin Meridian Group (Lateral)

THE URINARY BLADDER meridian begins at the inner corner of the eye and ascends to the occiput at the top of the head. It then descends lateral to the spine, over the sacrum, and down the posterior aspect of the leg to the back of the knee. It jumps to the top of the back, lateral to its previous line down the spinal column, passing the medial border of the scapula. It travels down the back, over the gluteus muscles, past the knee and down the back of the leg. It curves between the malleolus and the Achilles tendon, descending the lateral side of the foot, ending beside the nail of the little toe.

as a shield when we are afraid. The Urinary Bladder meridian often takes the brunt of the emotional pain that we are unwilling to experience and work through. Instead, the pain becomes stuck in the body and manifests as chronic pain.

Harmony
> willingness to confront emotional pain
> healthy urination

Disharmony
> frequent urination
> burning, painful, bloody, or urgent urination
> dark, scanty urination
> turbid urine
> chronic cystitis
> back pain
> acting "defensive"
> excessive suspicion of others
> sciatica

Kidney & Urinary Bladder Meridian Groups Asanas
Strength

For living without fear, relieving back pain, aiding in healthy urination, and opening up to the possibility of conquering chronic illness and pain. Accessing inner will-power.

PERICARDIUM AND TRIPLE BURNER

Pericardium

Although the pericardium is, anatomically, merely a membranous sac that surrounds the heart, in TCM the Pericardium is considered a separate organ than the Heart. However, the physiological functions and emotional manifestations of the Pericardium and Heart are similar. In TCM, the Pericardium is conceptualized as the "heart protector," as it encapsulates the Heart, shielding it from pathogens.

The Pericardium's emotional manifestation is *intimacy*. In TCM, the Heart is seen as an emperor, and the Pericardium is the emperor's most trusted guard. The Pericardium is the last defense before the Heart, and so its duty is to decide who will be allowed into the inner chambers of the Self. Disharmonies of the Pericardium may be similar to that of the Heart (insomnia, anxiety), but can also include fear of intimacy on the one hand, and overly permissive and inappropriate intimacy on the other.

In general, Pericardium disharmonies are similar to Heart disharmonies, with the addition of more physical channel pain around the chest and down the arm.

Harmony
>appropriate emotional engagement with others
>healthy mental-emotional state

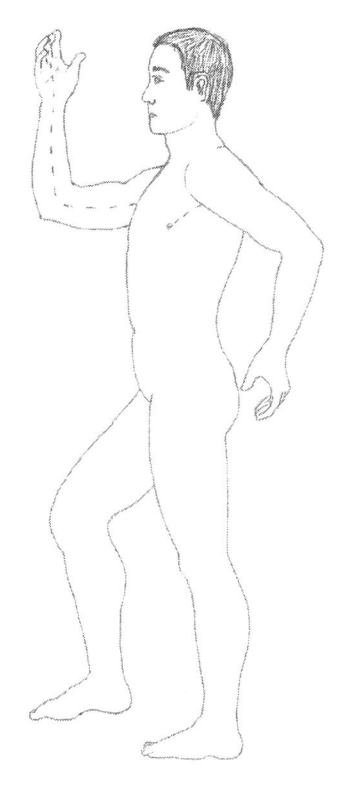

Three Arm Yin Meridian Group

THE PERICARDIUM meridian begins beside the nipple. It extends down the anterior aspect of the arm, past the elbow, down the middle of the forearm between the two most visible tendons. It crosses the palm and ends at the tip of the middle finger.

Disharmony
> insomnia
> feeling of "oppression" or "stuffiness" in the chest
> shooting pain down the arm
> anxiety
> mental-emotional disorders
> problems with intimacy

Triple Burner

The Triple Burner (or San Jiao) is not an anatomical organ, but is instead the *relationship* between the organs. It is the communication necessary to keep the whole body functional. The Triple Burner regulates the movement of water (Yin) and metabolic fire (Yang), thus harmonizing the relationship between Yin and Yang. Most importantly, the Triple Burner *mobilizes Qi*, actively moving it between organs and differentiating the Qi within the organs to perform specific functions. While we can speak of the Qi of the entire body, we can also identify Spleen Qi, Lung Qi, Heart Qi, and so on. The Triple Burner allows the Qi to perform its various duties. The Triple Burner also regulates biorhythm, keeping the body in harmony with the ebb and flow of the day.

The Triple Burner is a system of three "burners," lower, middle, and upper. These burners can be seen as platforms for different activities. The lower burner is below the umbilicus, and encompasses the Liver, Kidneys, Urinary Bladder, Small Intestine, and Large

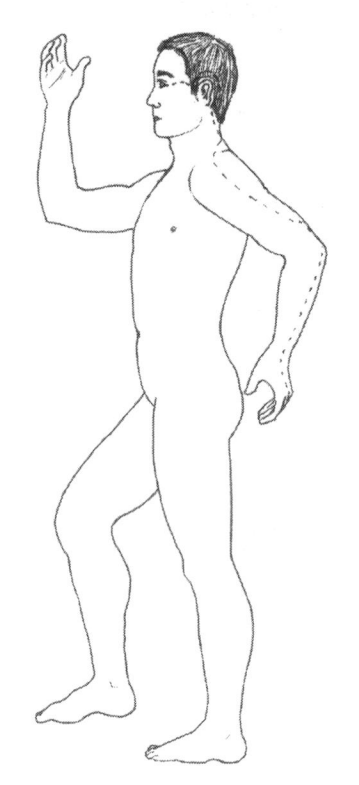

Three Arm Yang Meridian Group (Lateral)

THE TRIPLE BURNER meridian begins beside the nail of the ring finger. It extends over the dorsum of the hand and up the lateral aspect of the arm, between the radius and the ulna. It goes above the elbow and extends up the arm to the shoulder. It runs up the neck, around the ear, and ends at the lateral end of the eyebrow.

Intestine. It is the platform for sexual activity and the excretory part of the digestive process. The middle burner is between the diaphragm and umbilicus, and includes the Stomach, Spleen, and Gallbladder. It is the platform for digestion. The upper burner is from the diaphragm upward, encompassing the Lungs, Heart, and Pericardium. It is the platform for respiration and cardiac function. In each of the platforms, the Triple Burner mobilizes Qi, circulating metabolic fire (Yang) and fluids (Yin).

The Triple Burner and the Pericardium can be understood not as physical organs, but as *mediators*. The Pericardium mediates between the outside world and the Heart, and the Triple Burner mediates between the various organs of the body.

Harmony
> healthy metabolism and temperature regulation
> each of the component parts of the organ system works dynamically together as a whole

Disharmony
> edema
> problems with temperature regulation
> lack of communication and cooperation between organs

Pericardium & Triple Burner Meridian Groups Asanas
Harmony
For mediating relationships between self and others, allowing proper intimacy, regulating metabolism, and mobilizing the whole body to work in unity

LIVER AND GALLBLADDER

Liver

The Liver's most important function is storing Blood. It regulates the volume of Blood in the body, which influences energy levels. When there is not enough Blood in the body (in extreme cases, anemia), an individual may feel tired and depleted. The Liver also regulates menstruation; problems with menstruation (scanty, irregular, heavy, clotted, or painful menses) can almost always be traced back to the health of the Liver. Healthy menstruation, conception, and pregnancy depend on the Blood, and thus the Liver. Another function of the Liver Blood is to moisten the eyes and sinews (including tendons, ligaments, and cartilage). When there is insufficient Blood, the eyes may be dry and itchy, and the muscles may cramp.

The Liver's Blood also has an important effect on the Qi of the body. This reservoir of Blood is necessary to balance the Qi of the body—since Qi is Yang in nature and Blood is Yin, the two must keep a dynamic balance in order for the body to function properly. It's the Liver's job to make sure that Qi and Blood flow smoothly through the body.

The Liver is very important in maintaining overall emotional balance because of its relationship with Qi and Blood. In TCM, the Liver is understood as a

Anterior Thorax Meridian Group
Three Leg Yin Meridian Group (Medial)

THE LIVER meridian begins on the dorsal aspect of the big toe, beside the nail. It runs over the top of the foot, between the first and second toes. It continues up the medial aspect of the leg, past the crease of the groin, to the tip of the free end of the eleventh rib. It ends in the sixth intercostal space, in line with the nipple.

general of an army; it is an organ of *vision*, both physical (having to do with the eyes), as well as metaphorical: planning, foreseeing, and being assertive, while still being flexible. The Liver plans the body's functions by directing the Qi. When the Liver is healthy, the individual is relaxed and open to change, but is also able to assert oneself when necessary. When the Liver is in disharmony, we see frustration, anger, jealousy, agitation, feeling "trapped," poor vision, and menstrual problems. A person with a Liver imbalance will either express their anger in red-faced, explosive episodes, or they will hold their anger inside, feeling like it is inappropriate to express. It is often said say that depression is "anger turned inward," and indeed, this is seen with regard to the Liver. When the Liver is not permitted to channel its righteous anger outward, it instead turns this anger upon itself. This manifests as anxiety or depression.

In essence, the Liver's duty is to harmonize and balance—between Qi and Blood, and between decisive action and flexibility.

Harmony

emotional flexibility	foresight and good planning
assertiveness	ability to express healthy anger
good vision	regular and pain-free menstrual cycles

Disharmony

migraines	dysmenorrhea (painful menses)
muscle cramps	amenorrhea (absence of menses)
tremors or tics	pre-menstrual syndrome (PMS)
red, itchy eyes	feeling of a lump in the throat
blurred vision	irritability and frustration
poor night vision	explosive anger
dry skin and hair	anxiety or depression
jaundice	

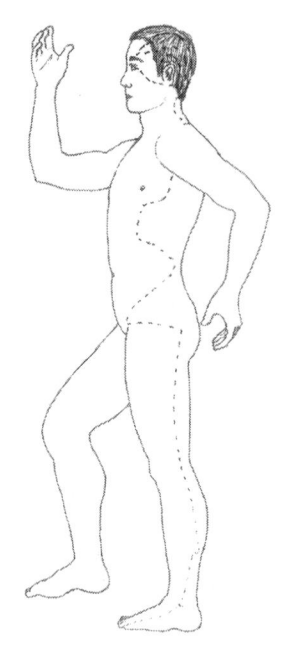

Lateral Thorax Meridian Group
Three Leg Yang Meridian Group (Lateral)

THE GALLBLADDER meridian begins lateral to the eye. It continues to the edge of the ear and flows up to a point at the side of the head. It curves back around the ear and then flows up to the scalp above the eye. It travels down to the forehead, then back to the scalp, curving around the skull to the back of the head.

The channel touches the crest of the trapezius muscle, and then moves down the side of the ribcage. It travels around the pelvic bone from the front to the back, and then moves down the lateral side of the leg. On the top of the foot, it runs between the fourth and fifth toes, ending beside the nail of the fourth toe.

Gallbladder

The Gallbladder stores and secretes bile, which assists the Spleen, Stomach, Small Intestine, and Large Intestine in the process of digestion. Emotionally, the Gallbladder corresponds to *courage* and *decision-making*. The Liver makes plans and the Gallbladder executes them. The Gallbladder actualizes and takes initiative; thus, a disharmony of the Gallbladder could show up as timidity or indecisiveness in the case of deficiency, or as recklessness and bullheadedness in the case of excess. Together, the Liver and Gallbladder help us make our way through the world, flexible as needed and decisive when the time is right.

Harmony
    healthy digestion
    strong decision-making
    courage

Disharmony
    genital rash and itching
    pain in the ribcage
    jaundice
    inability to digest fats
    cholelithiasis (gallstones)
    bitter taste in the mouth
    impulsivity
    irrational arguments
    stubbornness

Liver & Gallbladder Meridian Groups Asanas
Balance

For bringing the body back into balance, working through anger issues, detoxifying, regulating menstruation, and improving vision, creating ease and decisiveness.

THE GOVERNING AND CONCEPTION VESSELS

In addition to the twelve meridians associated with organs, there are also eight "extraordinary vessels," which are not associated with organs. These vessels/meridians are considered to be the first thing to develop in the fetus in the uterus, before the lungs or the heart, right when the zygote is formed and the cells are beginning to divide. These are the basic channels of our being. We will focus on two of the eight extraordinary vessels: The Governing Vessel and The Conception Vessel.

Governing Vessel

The Governing Vessel is known as the "Sea of Yang channels" because it influences and strengthens all the Yang channels of the body (Large Intestine, Stomach, Small Intestine, Triple Burner, and Gallbladder).

The Governing Vessel has four main functions. First, because of the trajectory of its channel, it can be used to strengthen the spine and back. It is especially useful in cases of chronic low back pain due to Kidney deficiency, as its channel runs between the kidneys and

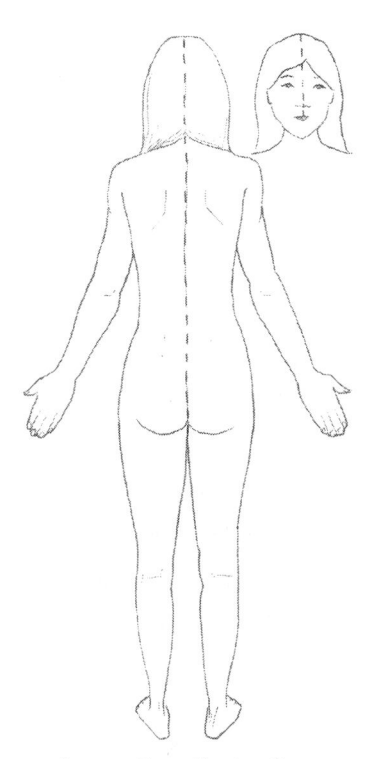

Posterior Thorax Meridian Group

THE GOVERNING VESSEL begins midway between the coccyx and the anus. It travels up the spine. It then curves around the skull at the midline, running down the forehead, over the tip of the nose and the upper lip, and ending at the tip of the upper lip.

along the spine. It can also be used to straighten the spine, in cases of scoliosis or poor posture.

Second, the Governing Vessel nourishes the brain. The channel goes up the back of the neck, over the skull, and ends at the upper lip, thus running over the top part of the head. In TCM, the brain contains Jing ("essence"); in order for the Jing to travel from the Kidneys to the brain, it must be carried by the Governing Vessel. The health of the brain depends on the Governing Vessel. The Governing Vessel therefore calms the mind and stimulates the memory.

Third, the Governing Vessel can be used to treat dizziness, convulsions, tremors, epilepsy, and the aftermath of stroke.

Fourth, because of the Yang quality of the channel, as well as its trajectory up the spine, the Governing Vessel has a lifting and energizing effect. Moods lift as Qi rises. Thus, the Governing Channel can be used to treat depression, as well as prolapse of organs. The Governing Vessel is very useful in treating emotional disorders. Emotionally, when the Governing Vessel is healthy, a person stands tall and confident, with a strong sense of self. On physical, emotional, and spiritual planes, the Governing Vessel encourages us to be *upright*.

Harmony
    healthy back, brain, and spine
    healthy sense of self

Disharmony

scoliosis	prolapse of organs (uterus, rectum)
low back pain	epilepsy, convulsions, tremors
depression	lack of confidence

Conception Vessel

The Conception Vessel is called the "Sea of all Yin channels," and strengthens the Yin of all the channels and organs, as well as the Fluids and Blood of the body. Its most important function is regulating the reproductive system of both men and women, as it travels over the genitals and also has a strong effect on the Kidneys. For women in particular, the Conception Vessel is of utmost importance in puberty, menstruation, fertility, conception, pregnancy, childbirth, and menopause.

Emotionally, the Conception Vessel corresponds to the health of our Yin. It reminds us to accept and embrace the people and the world around us. The health of both the Governing Vessel and the Conception Vessel as a pair is crucial for our emotional health—the Governing Vessel lets us rise up strongly (straightening the spine) as an individual with a destiny and personal truth, and the Conception Vessel lets us relax into community, oneness, and the realization that we are part of something larger than ourselves. While the Governing Vessel urges us to be upright, the Conception Vessel reminds us to be *compassionate*. This Yin-Yang dynamic is the crux of our emotional health.

Harmony
    healthy reproductive function
    acceptance of self and others

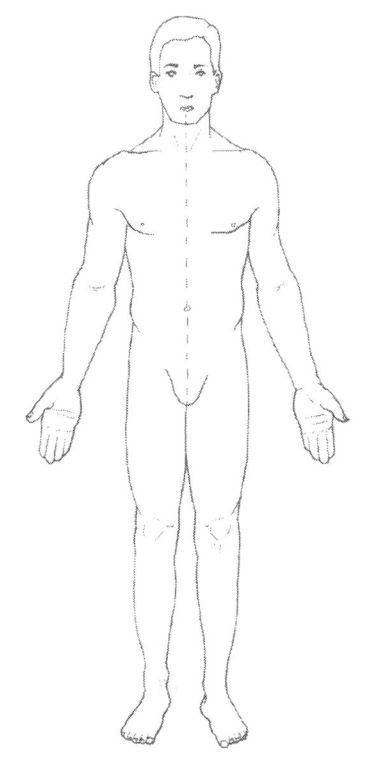

Anterior Thorax Meridian Group

THE CONCEPTION VESSEL starts at the perineum. It travels up through the front midline of the body and ends between the chin and the lower lip.

Disharmony
> difficult puberty and menstruation
> menopausal syndrome
> infertility

Governing Vessel & Conception Vessel Meridian Groups Asanas
Truth

For emotional balance, an understanding of one's personal truths and one's place in the greater whole, for fertility, and for spinal issues.

CHAPTER 9

Meridian Groups

THE YOGA ASANAS AND SEQUENCES in this book are designed to stimulate Qi flow and remove Qi blockages of different groups of meridians, according to their location and pathways throughout the body. Unlike acupuncture, it is nearly impossible to target single meridians through a yoga practice. Yoga asanas manipulate whole body regions that include several different meridians. The meridian groups are as follows:

MERIDIANS	MERIDIAN GROUPS
Lungs, Pericardium, Stomach, Liver, Kidney, Conception Vessel	Anterior Thorax
Spleen, Gallbladder	Lateral Thorax
Urinary Bladder, Governing Vessel	Posterior Thorax
Heart, Pericardium, Lung	Three Arm Yin (medial)
Small Intestine, Triple Burner Large Intestine	Three Arm Yang (lateral)
Spleen, Liver, Kidney	Three Leg Yin (medial)
Stomach, Urinary Bladder Gallbladder	Tree Leg Yang (lateral)

CHAPTER 10

Designing your practice

THIS BOOK IS DESIGNED to help you tailor the yoga practice that best fits your needs and improve your physical and emotional well-being. In the previous chapters, identify the meridians and organ's functions which you wish to balance and harmonize. Continue by locating the meridian groups that include your designated meridians and partner organs. Finally, choose the asanas and asana sequences that target the specific meridian groups.

Vary Your Practice

Experiment with various asanas and asana sequences. All of the asanas in this book are beneficial. However, different asanas at different times may better work for you. Practice the asanas that are designed to harmonize your specific physical and/or emotional needs and concerns. However, avoid practicing only a single set of asanas over a long period of time. Instead, alternate between the different meridian groups asanas and asana sequences and make sure not to neglect practicing asanas of any meridian group.

Length of Holding the Poses

The asanas should be held between thirty to forty seconds, according to your needs. Experiment staying in the various asanas for different lengths of time and see how they make you feel. Whatever you choose, it is important to avoid staying in the asanas too long or overextending yourself. The entire practice should remain at your comfort level while pushing yourself just a little bit more each time.

Breath

While practicing Meridian Systems Yoga, the breath should be slightly longer and slightly deeper than your ordinary breath. Try to use the breath to further stretch and elongate the body. As you inhale, imagine the breath starting at the sacrum and traveling up through the spine and the Governing Vessel all the way to the top of the head. With every breath allow the entire back to grow longer and wider. Exhale through the Conception Vessel, on the front side of the body. Starting from the top of the head, move down over the nose, through the neck and chest, over the umbilicus, ending in the perineum.

This breathing sequence, up the Governing Vessel and down the Conception Vessel, is a powerful practice of harmonizing the Yin and Yang of the body. Similarly, move through the limbs, making them longer and wider with every breath. Inhale from the tips of the toes of one leg, moving to the fingers tips of the opposite hand. In the next breath, start at the tips of the toes of the other leg, ending at the finger tips of the opposite hand. While practicing, try to alternate between breathing up the Governing Vessel and down the Conception Vessel, and breathing through the limbs. Whatever you choose, make sure not to overdo it. The breath should always remain gentle. Breathing too much or to hard my cause hyperventilation and discomfort.

Length of practice

A practice may take anywhere between fifteen to forty minutes, depending on the amount of time and energy you have. It is important not to neglect or overdo your practice. Neglecting your practice will not allow you to achieve the benefits of this method. Over-practicing can create a burden that may result in you giving up yoga altogether. At times, you may practice just a couple of asanas to help you better deal with stress or tension. Several asanas could be practiced literally anywhere. For example, see Gomukhasana arm using a chair (page 73)

Day, Times and Frequency of Practice

Try alternating your practice between first thing in the morning, during the day, or when you arrive back at home in the evening. An early morning practice will give you energy and a sense of peace and harmony to carry out your affairs throughout the day. An afternoon practice will help you overcome tiredness and maintain a positive attitude for the rest of your work day. An evening practice will help you relax and move through various emotions and stressors (stimulating Qi flow and removing Qi blockages) that were acquired during the day. It will also help you sleep better throughout the night.

Whenever you practice, it should always feel comfortable. Trying too hard to establish and maintain a practice could lead to failure. Thus, it is important to experiment practicing the different yoga asanas and asana sequences at different times of the day. Discover what feels best and what brings forth best results.

Location for your practice

Designate a comfortable, clean, and quiet place at home for your practice. Make sure there is enough open space so you may freely practice without the risk of bumping into furniture. Having a designated place that you like coming back to will also help you maintain your practice. Over time, it may become a sacred place for you, a place for balancing, unwinding, and rejoicing.

Meridian Systems Yoga Asanas

The asanas in the following chapters are divided into their perspective meridian groups. Additional meridian groups are presented next to each asana that stimulates more than one anatomical region.

CHAPTER 11

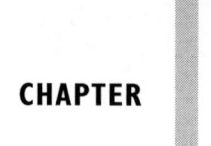

Meridian Systems Yoga Asanas

ANTERIOR THORAX MERIDIAN GROUP ASANAS

Pericardium, Lung, Stomach, Liver, Kidney, Conception Vessel

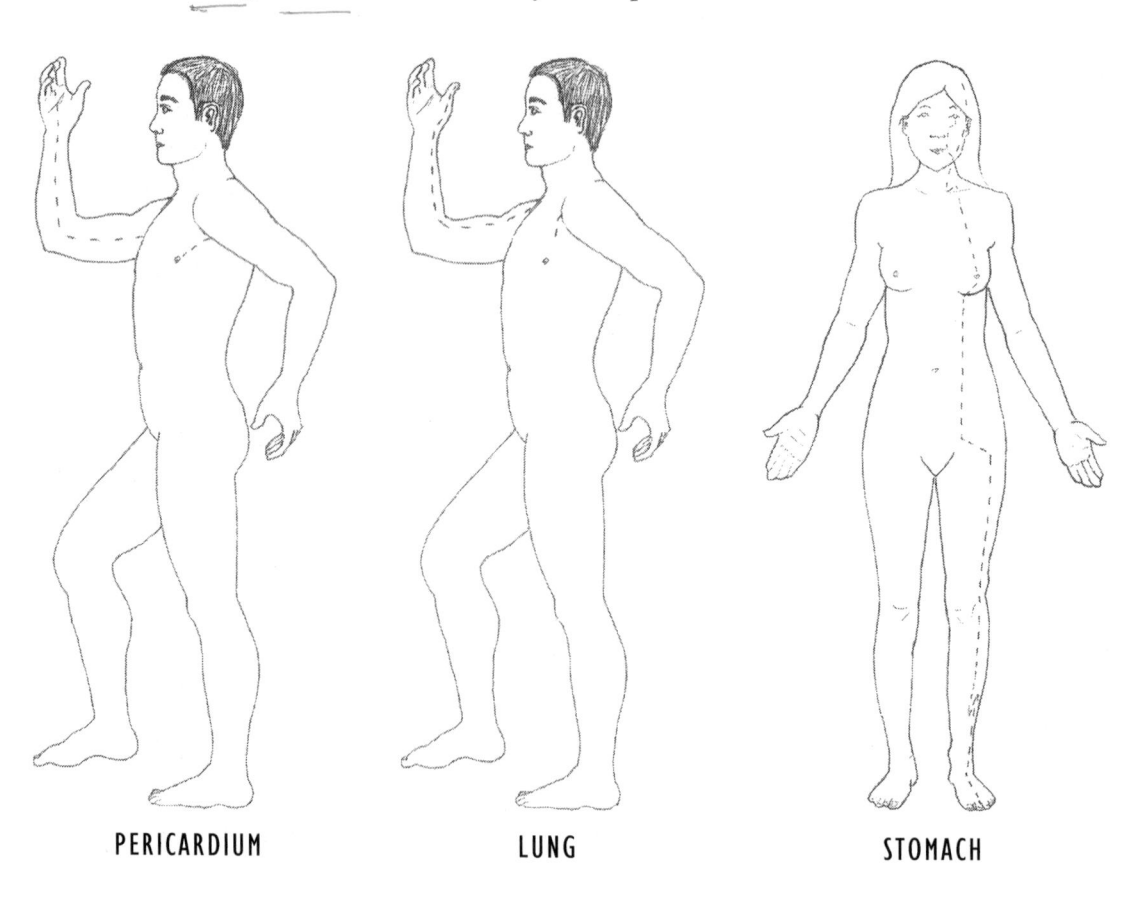

PERICARDIUM   LUNG   STOMACH

Meridian Systems Yoga Asanas 47

LIVER   KIDNEY   CONCEPTION VESSEL

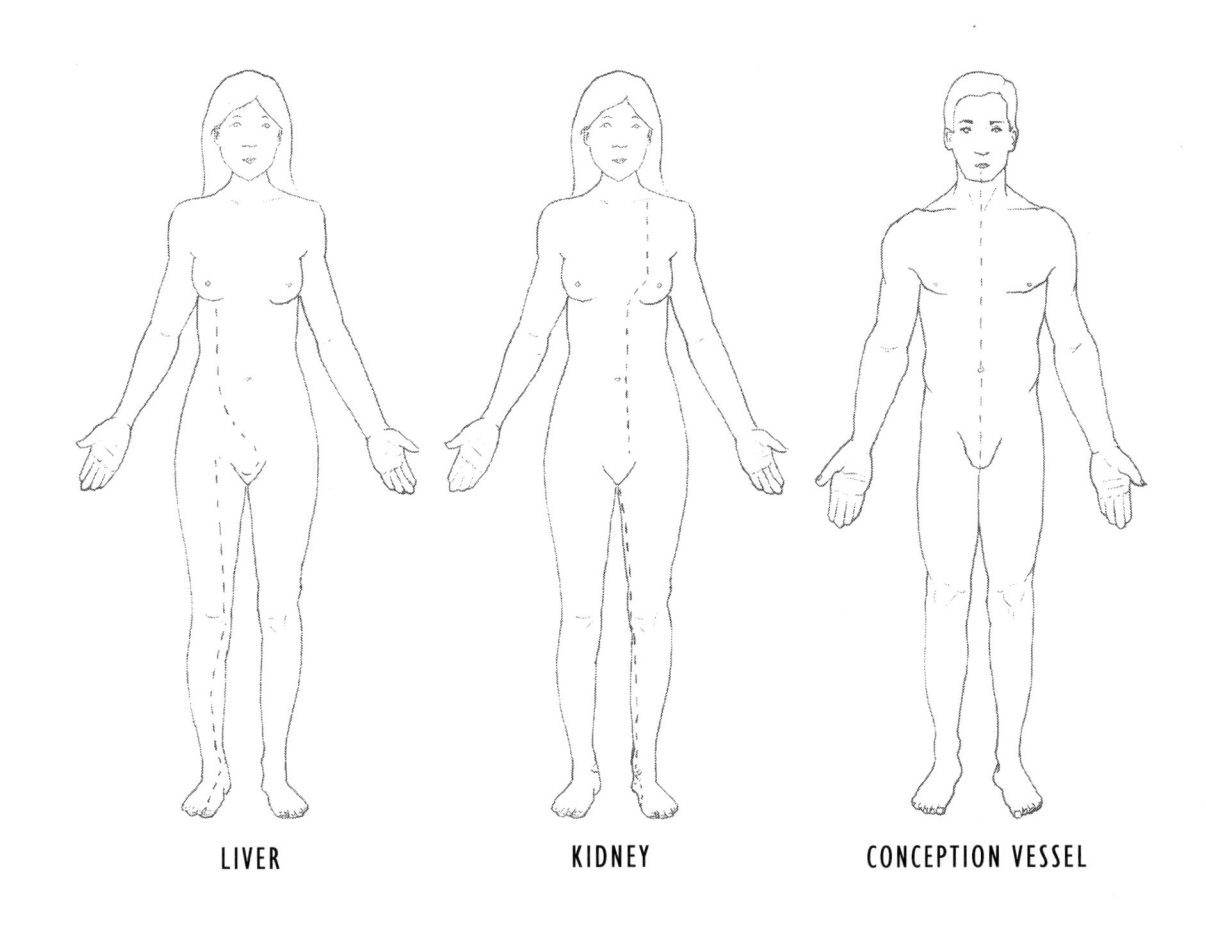

Anterior Thorax

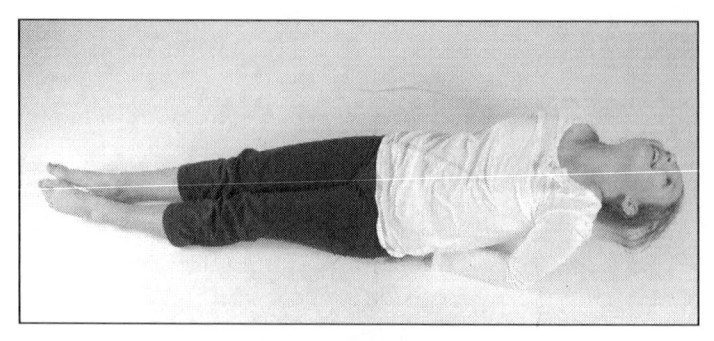

Matsyasana — Fish Pose

Also Stimulates the Following:

Three Leg Yin
Three Leg Yang
Three Arm Yin
Three Arm Yang

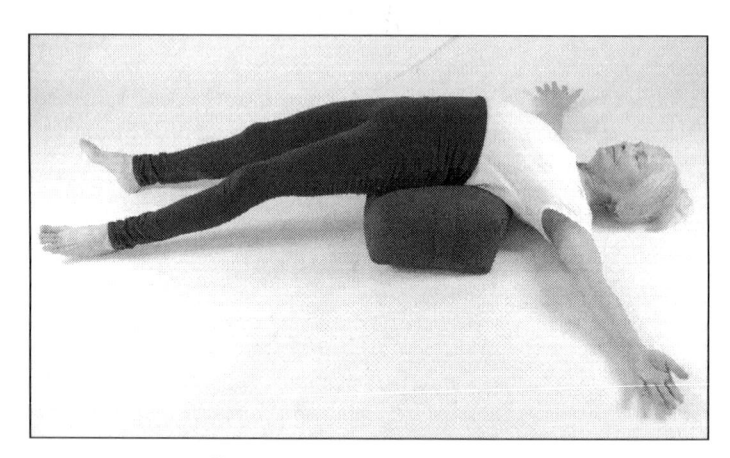

Matsyasana on a Bolster — Fish Pose

Anterior Thorax 49

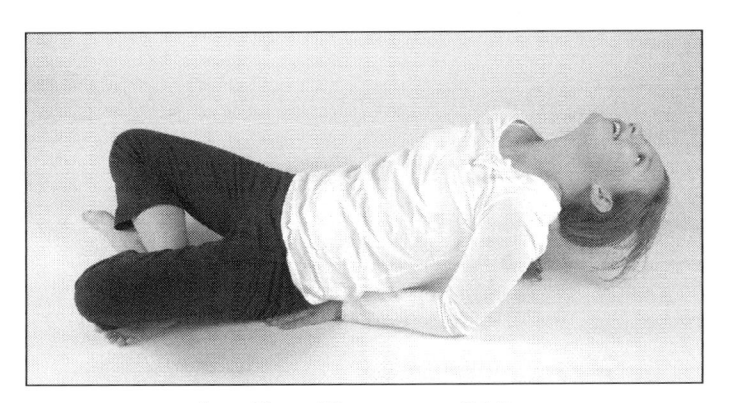

Crossed Legged Matsyasana — Fish Pose

Also Stimulates the Following:

Three Leg Yin
Three Leg Yang

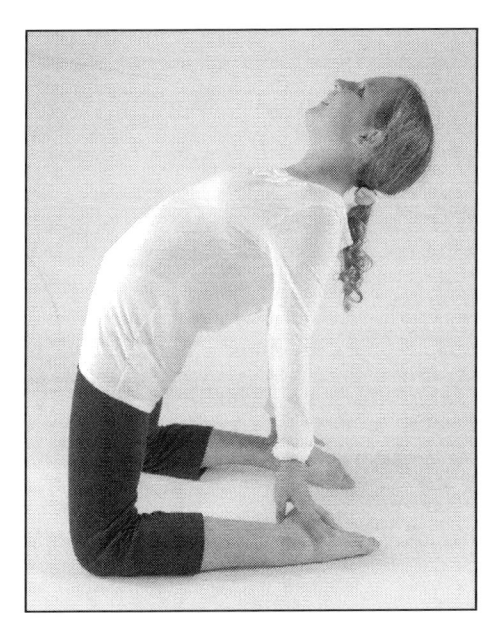

Ustrasana — Camel Pose

Also Stimulates the Following:

Three Arm Yin
Three Arm Yang
Three Leg Yin
Three Leg Yang

Anterior Thorax *continued*

Also Stimulates the Following:

Three Arm Yin
Three Arm Yang
Three Leg Yin
Three Leg Yang

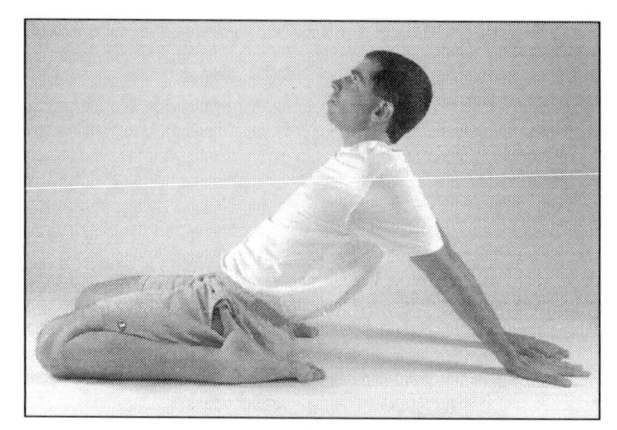

Ardha Supta Virasana — Half Reclining Hero Pose

Also Stimulates the Following:

Three Arm Yin
Three Arm Yang
Lateral Thorax
Three Leg Yang

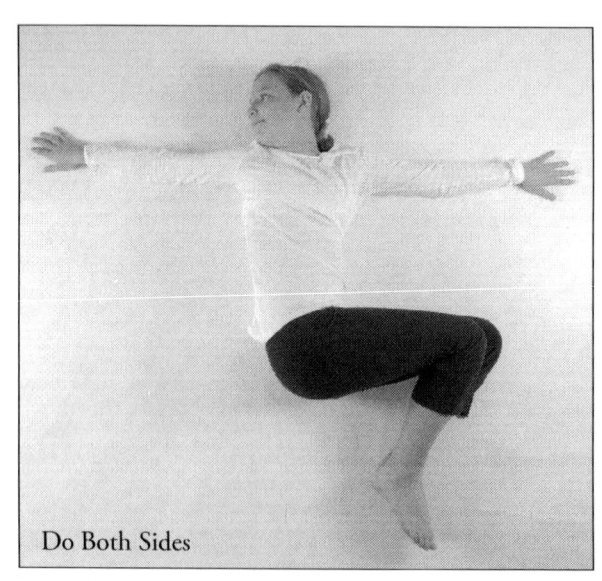

Do Both Sides

Supta Parivrtta Balasana — Reclining Child's Pose

Do Both Sides

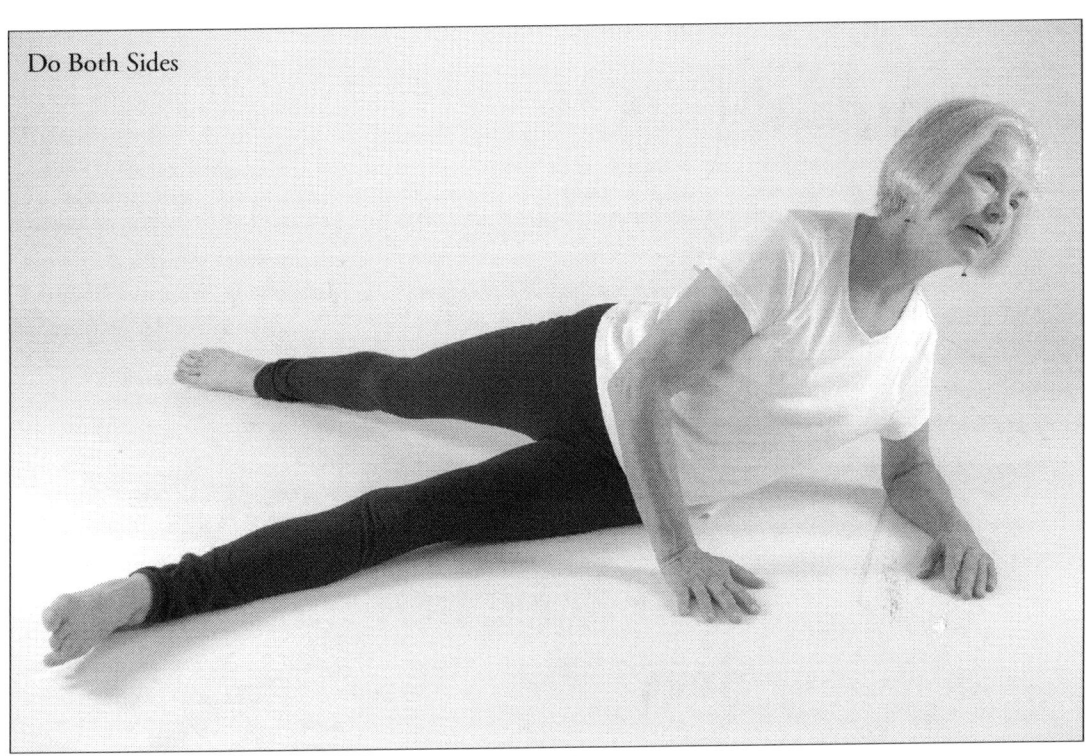

Supta Parivrtta Upavistha Konasana I —
Reclined revolved wide-angle seated forward bend

Also Stimulates the Following:

Lateral Thorax
Posterior Thorax
Three Leg Yin
Three Leg Yang

Anterior Thorax *continued*

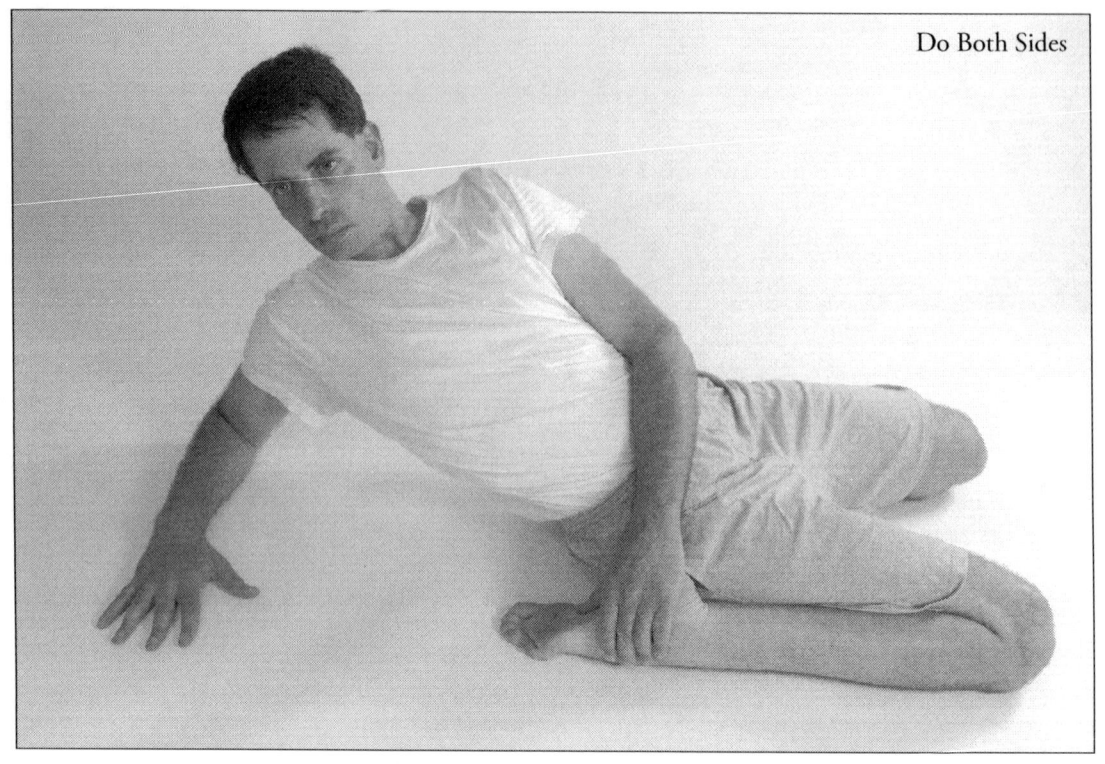

Do Both Sides

Parivrtta Ardha Supta Virasana I – Half Reclining Hero Pose

Also Stimulates the Following:

Lateral Thorax
Three Leg Yin
Three Leg Yang

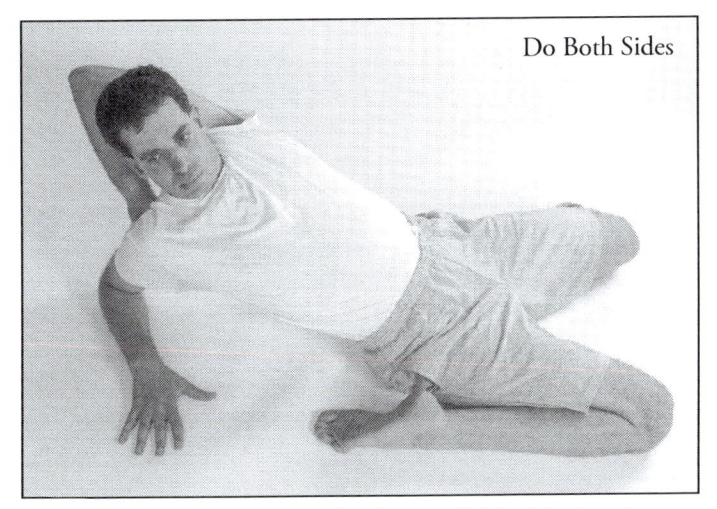

Anterior Thorax   53

Do Both Sides

Parivrtta Ardha Supta Virasana II — Revolved Half Reclining Hero Pose

Back View

Also Stimulates the Following:

Three Arm Yin   Autumn
Three Arm Yang
Three Leg Yin
Three Leg Yang

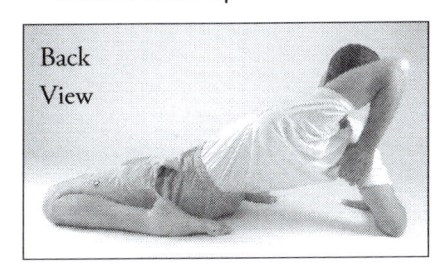

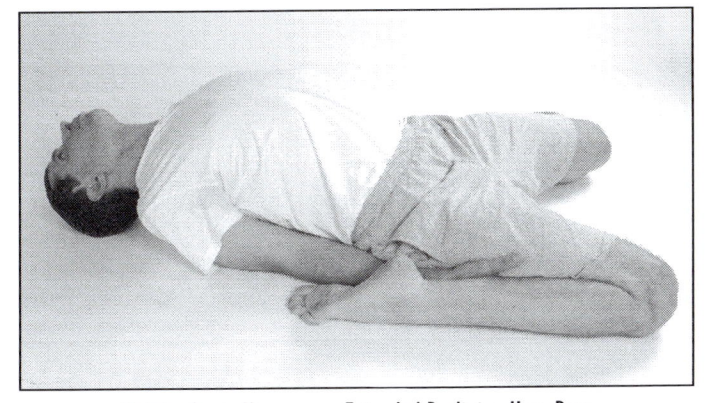

Utthita Supta Virasana — Extended Reclining Hero Pose

Also Stimulates the Following:

Three Leg Yin
Three Leg Yang

LATERAL THORAX MERIDIAN GROUP ASANAS

Spleen and Gallbladder

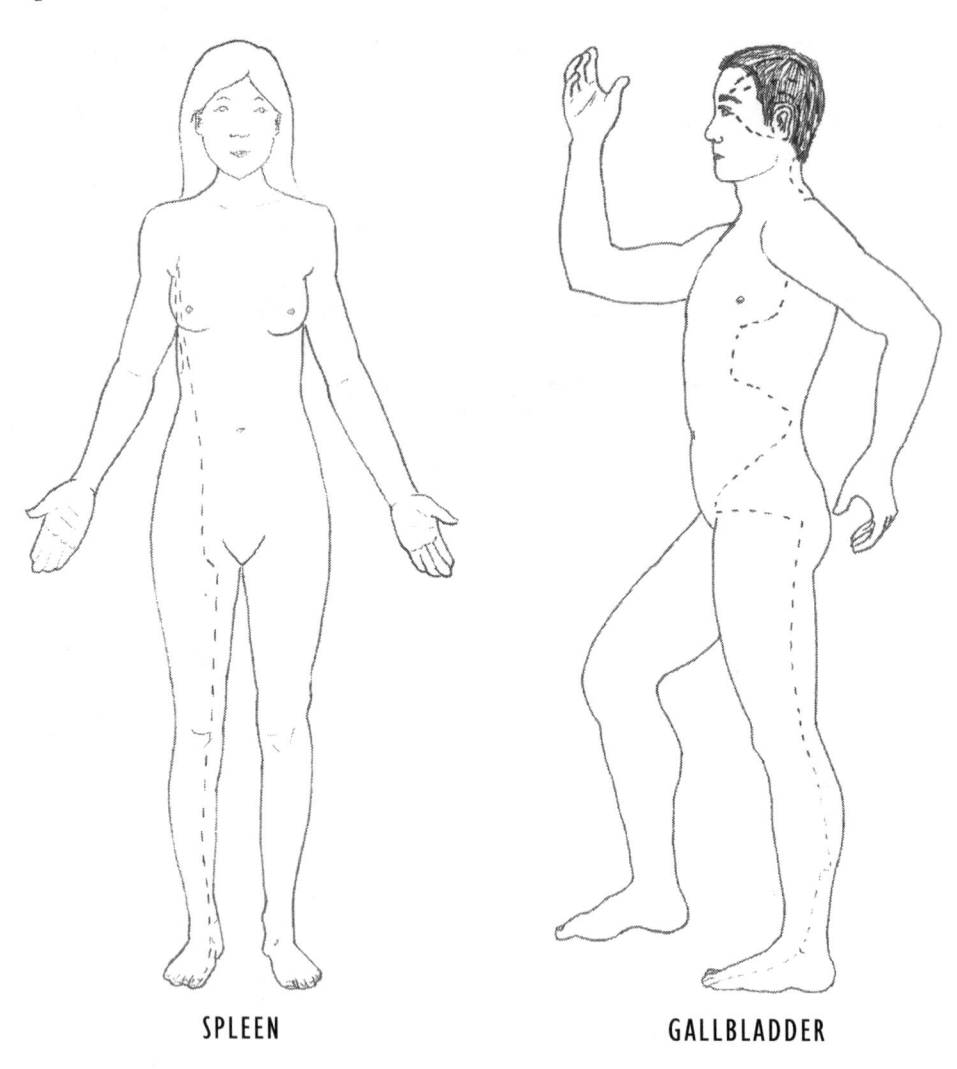

SPLEEN   GALLBLADDER

Lateral Thorax

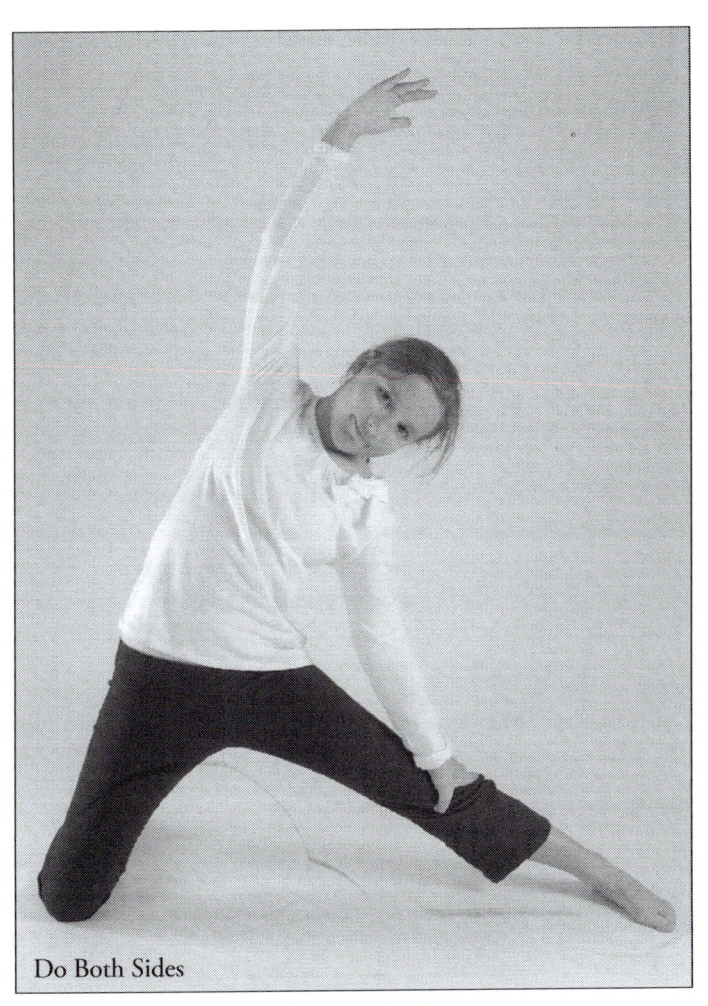

Also Stimulates the Following:

Three Leg Yin
Three Leg Yang
Three Arm Yang Autumn

Do Both Sides

Parighasana — Gate Pose

Lateral Thorax *continued*

Also Stimulates the Following:

Posterior Thorax

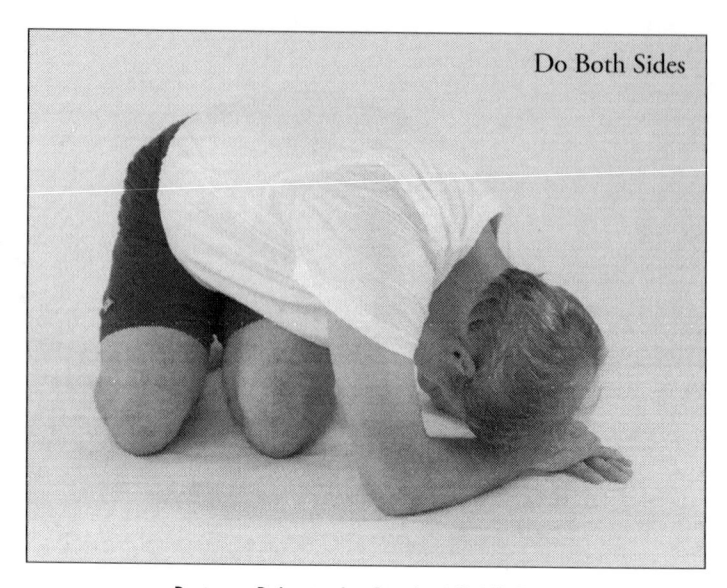

Parivrtta Balasana I — Revolved Child's Pose

Also Stimulates the Following:

Posterior Thorax

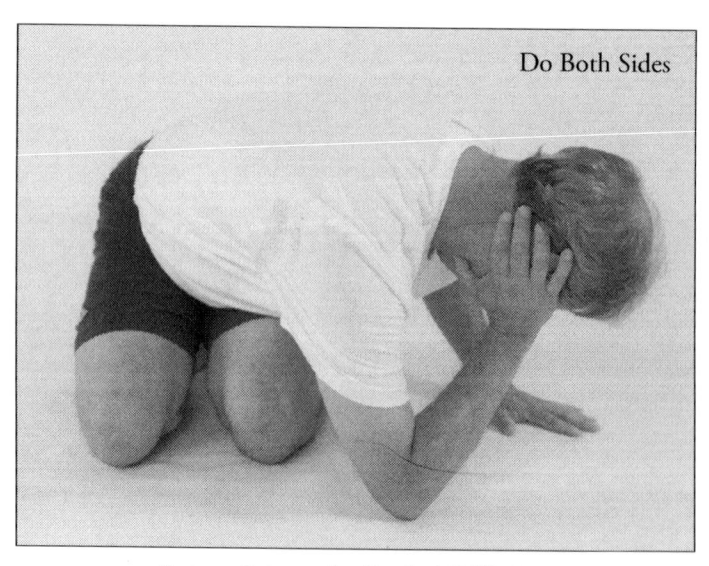

Parivrtta Balasana II — Revolved Child's Pose

Lateral Thorax   57

Do Both Sides

Lateral Stretch

Also Stimulates the Following:

Three Leg Yang
Three Arm Yang

58 Meridian Systems Yoga

Lateral Thorax *continued*

Also Stimulates the Following:

Anterior Thorax A
Posterior Thorax
Three Leg Yin
Three Leg Yang

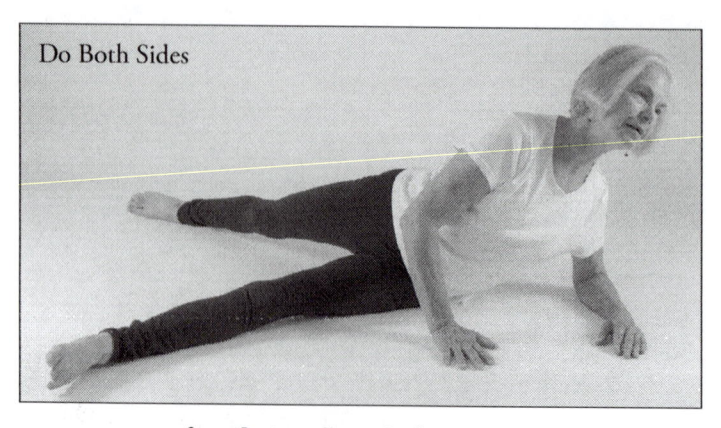

Do Both Sides

Supta Parivrtta Upavistha Konasana I —
Reclining revolved wide-angle seated forward bend

Also Stimulates the Following:

Anterior Thorax A
Posterior Thorax
Three Leg Yin
Three Leg Yang

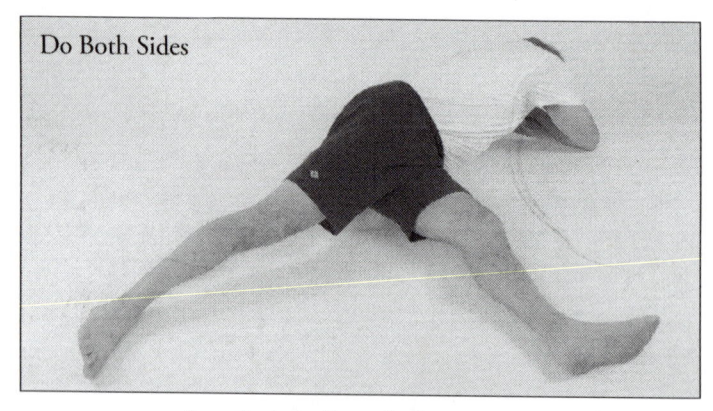

Do Both Sides

Supta Parivrtta Upavistha Konasana II —
Reclining revolved wide-angle seated forward bend

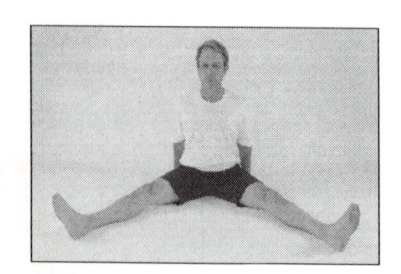

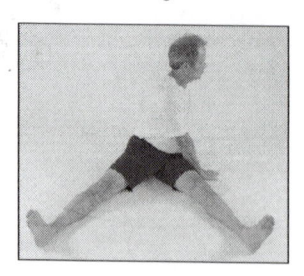

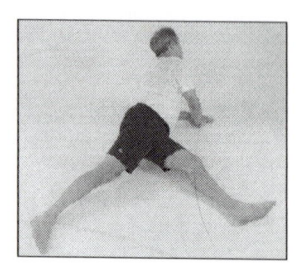

Lateral Thorax 59

Also Stimulates the Following:

Anterior Thorax Autumn
Posterior Thorax

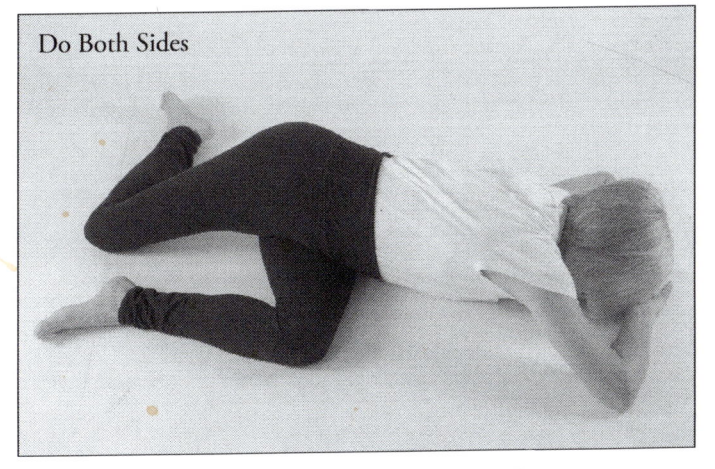

Do Both Sides

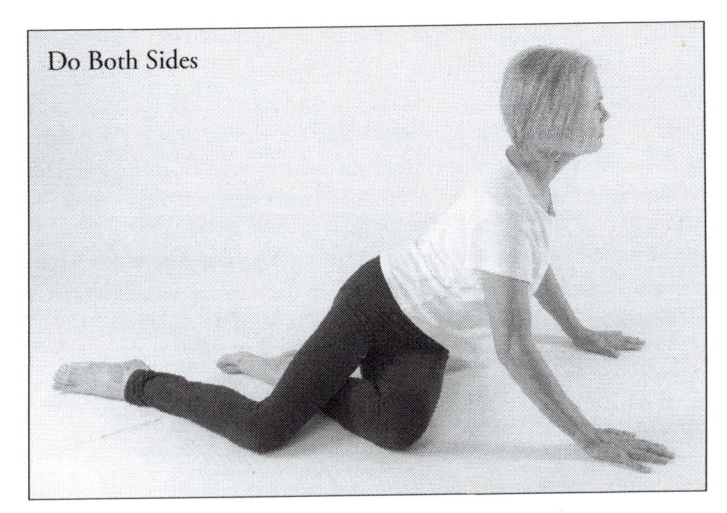

Supta Bharadvajasana I — Bharadvaja's Twist

Also Stimulates the Following:

Posterior Thorax

Do Both Sides

Supta Bharadvajasana II — Bharadvaja's Twist

Lateral Thorax *continued*

Also Stimulates the Following:

Posterior Thorax
Three Arm Yin A
Three Arm Yang A

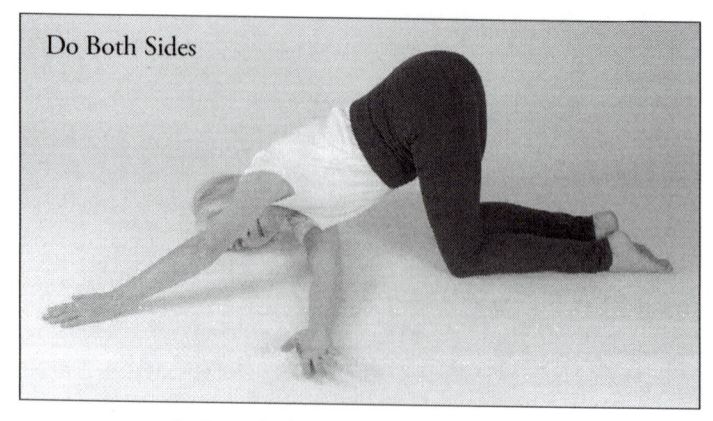

Parivrtta Bitilasana I — Revolved Cow Pose

Also Stimulates the Following:

Posterior Thorax
Three Arm Yin
Three Arm Yang 3A

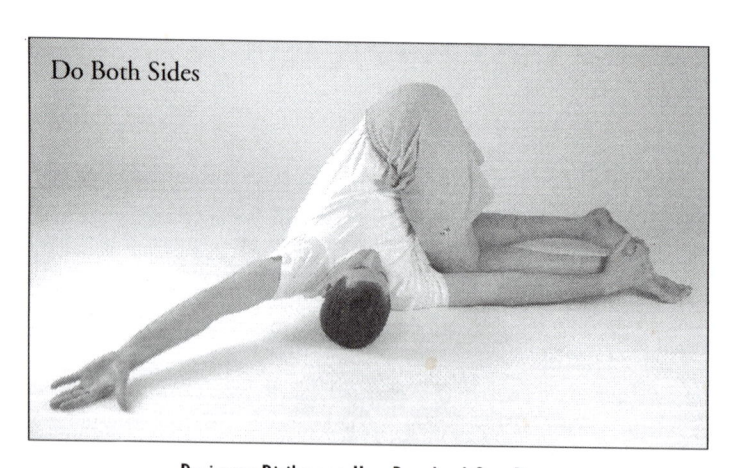

Parivrtta Bitilasana II — Revolved Cow Pose

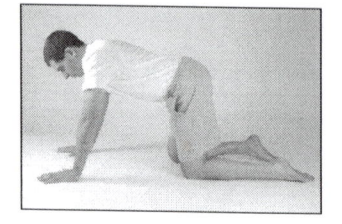

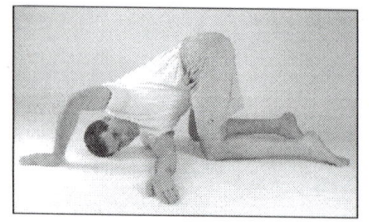

Do Both Sides

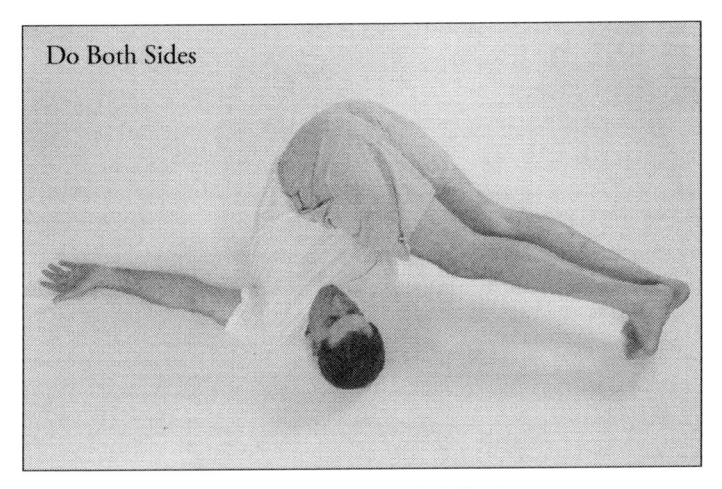

Parivrtta Halasana — Revolved Plow Pose

Also Stimulates the Following:

Posterior Thorax
Three Arm Yin
Three Arm Yang
Three Leg Yang

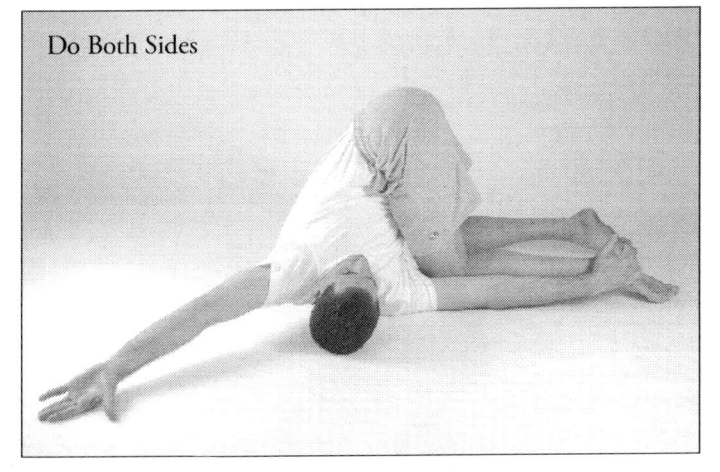

Do Both Sides

Parivrtta Bitilasana II - Revolved cow pose

Also Stimulates the Following:

Posterior Thorax
Three Arm Yin
Three Arm Yang
Three Leg Yang

Lateral Thorax *continued*

Also Stimulates the Following:

Posterior Thorax
Three Arm Yin
Three Leg Yin
Three Leg Yang

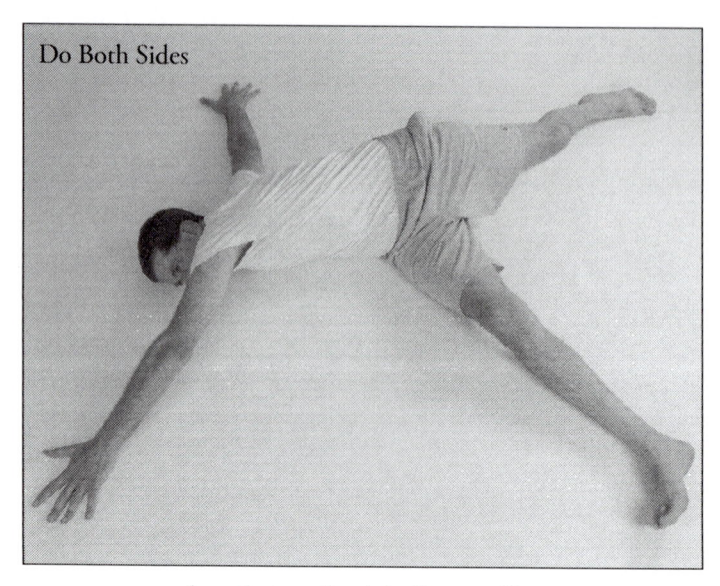

Do Both Sides

Supta Parivrtta Upavistha Konasana III—
Reclining Revolved Wide Angle Seated Forward Bend

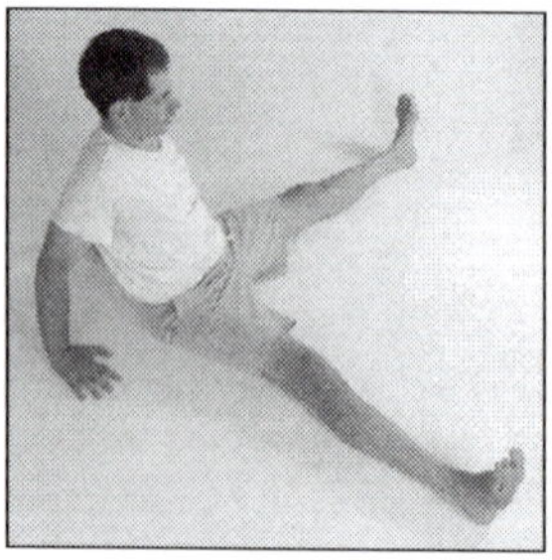

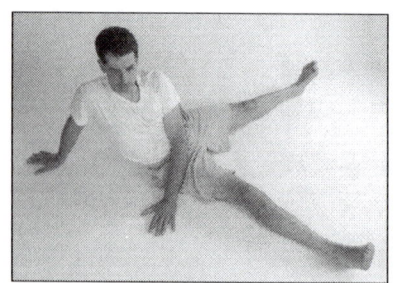

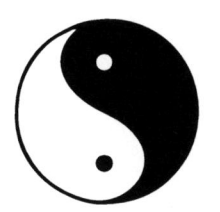

POSTERIOR THORAX MERIDIAN GROUP ASANAS

Urinary Bladder and Governing Vessel

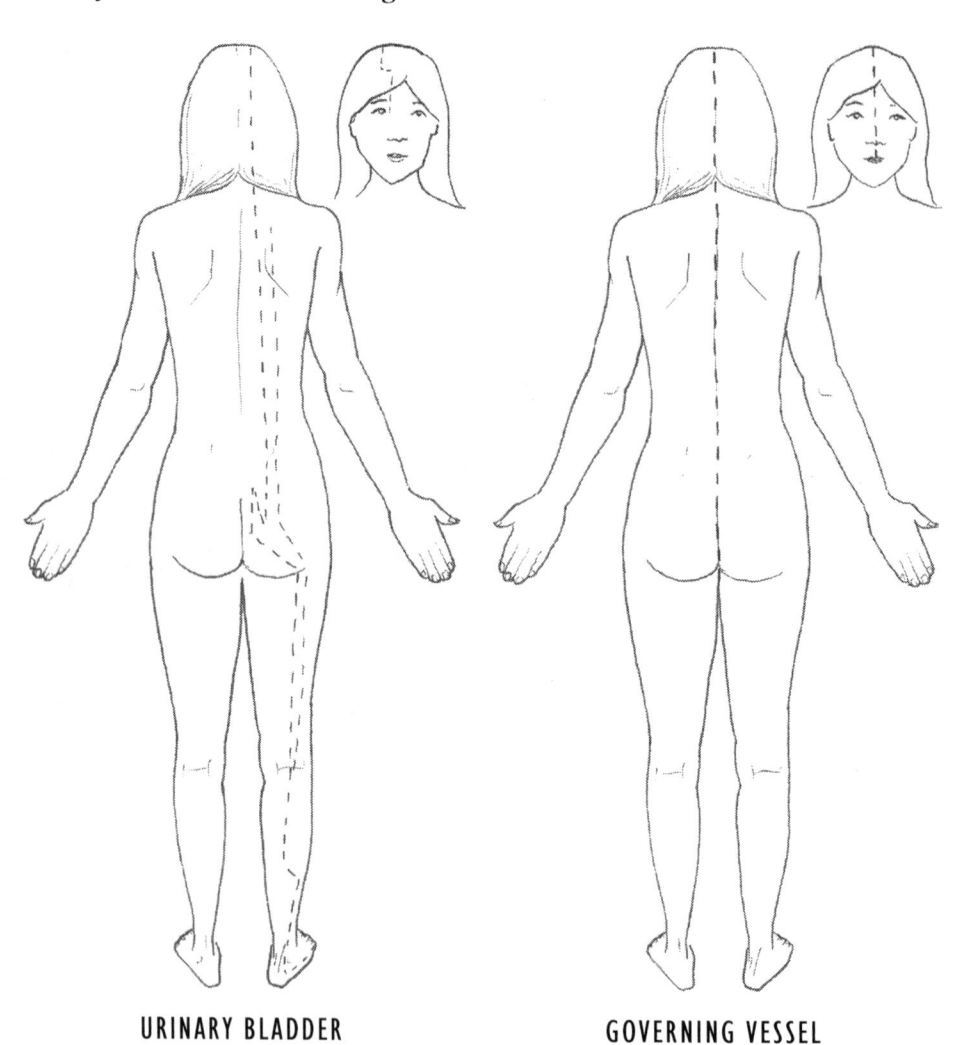

URINARY BLADDER

GOVERNING VESSEL

Posterior Thorax

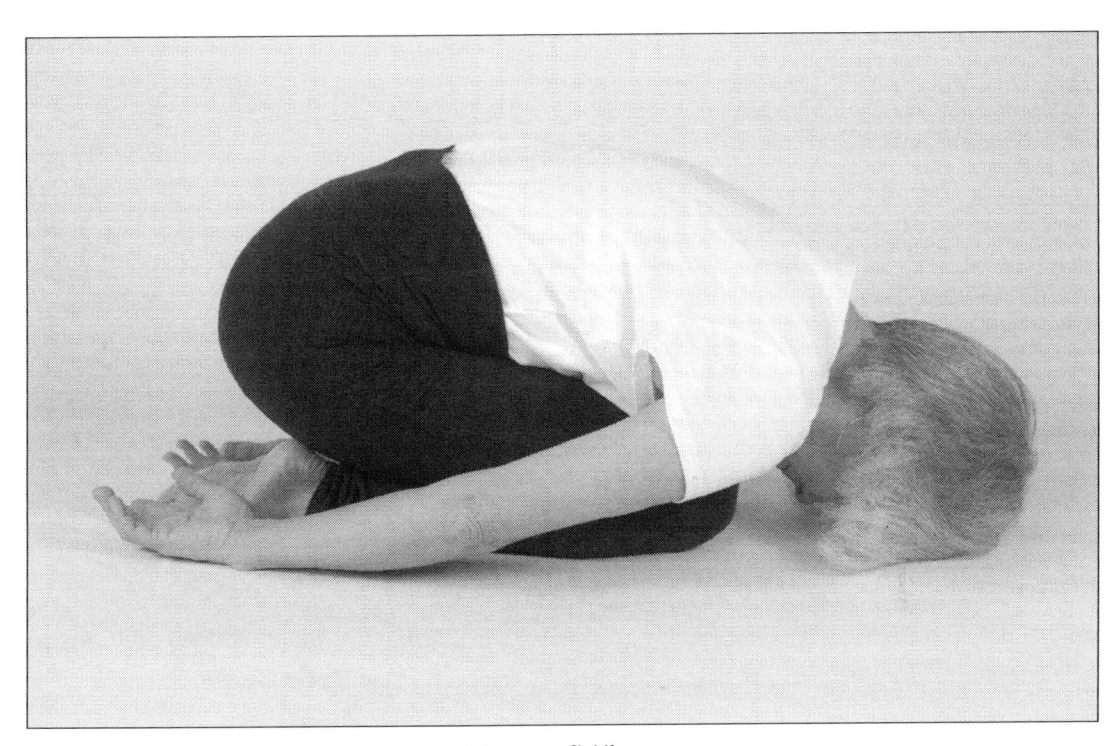

Balasana – Child's pose

Posterior Thorax *continued*

Also Stimulates the Following:

Three Leg Yin
Three Leg Yang

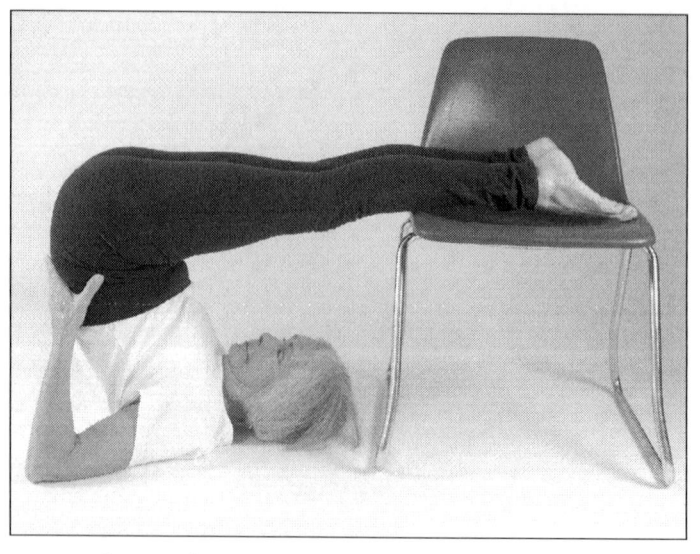

Prasarita Svanasana with Chair — Wide Legged Dog Pose

Also Stimulates the Following:

Three Leg Yin
Three Leg Yang
Three Arm Yang
Three Arm Yin

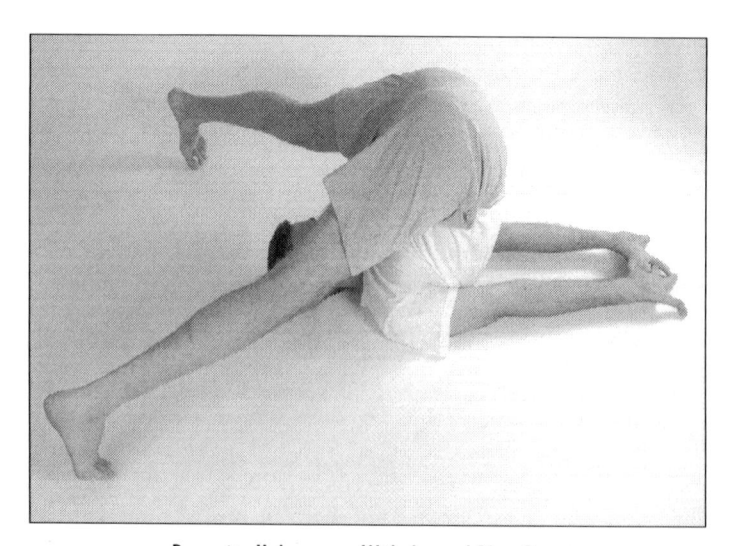

Prasarita Halasana — Wide Legged Plow Pose

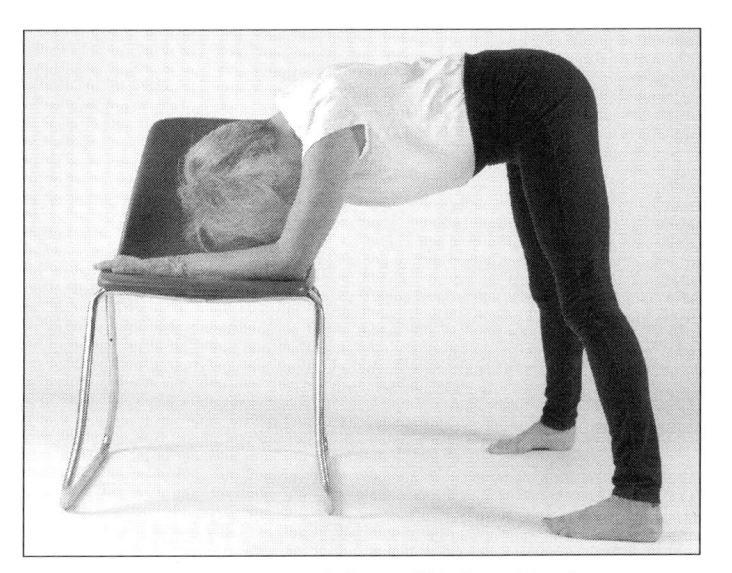

Posterior Thorax 67

Also Stimulates the Following:

Three Leg Yin
Three Leg Yang

Prasarita Svanasana with Chair — Wide Legged Dog Pose

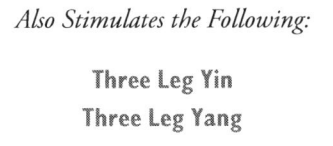

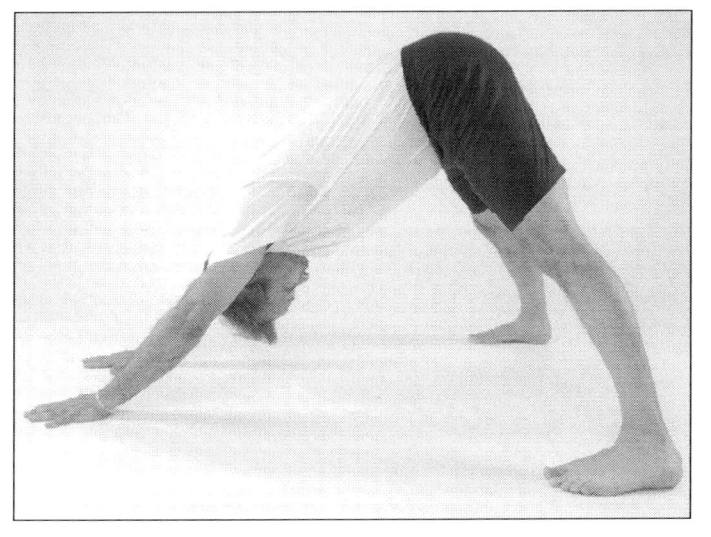

Also Stimulates the Following:

Three Leg Yin
Three Leg Yang

Prasarita Svanasana — Wide Legged Dog Pose

THREE ARM YIN AND THREE ARM YANG MERIDIAN GROUP ASANAS

Lungs and Large Intestines, Heart and Small Intestines, Pericardium and Triple Burner

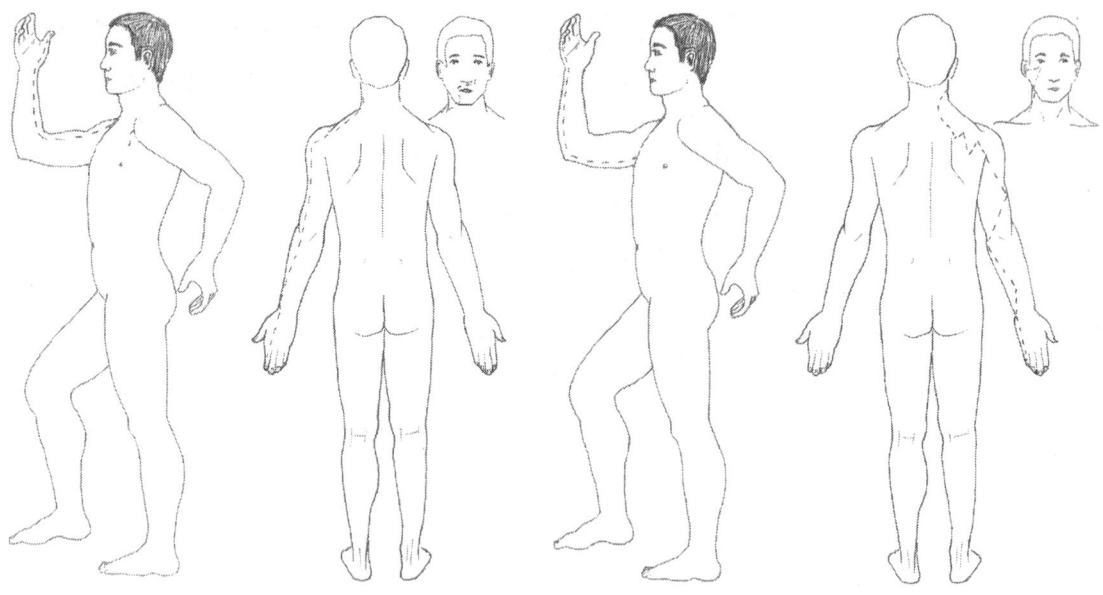

LUNGS AND LARGE INTESTINES

HEART AND SMALL INTESTINES

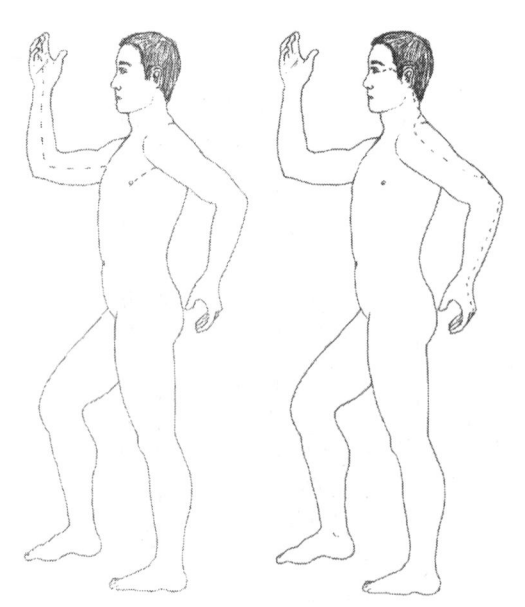

PERICARDIUM AND TRIPLE BURNER

Three Arm Yin and Three Arm Yang

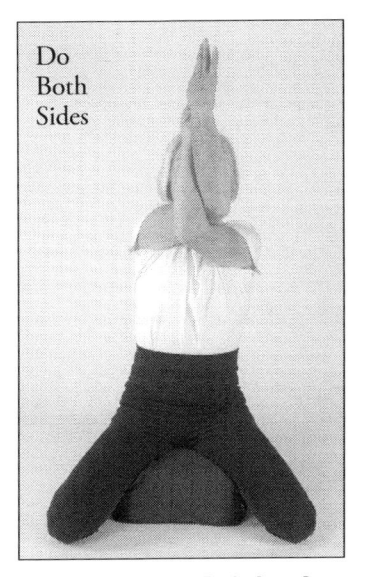

Garudasana Arms — Eagle Arms Pose

Also Stimulates the Following:

Three Leg Yin
Three Leg Yang

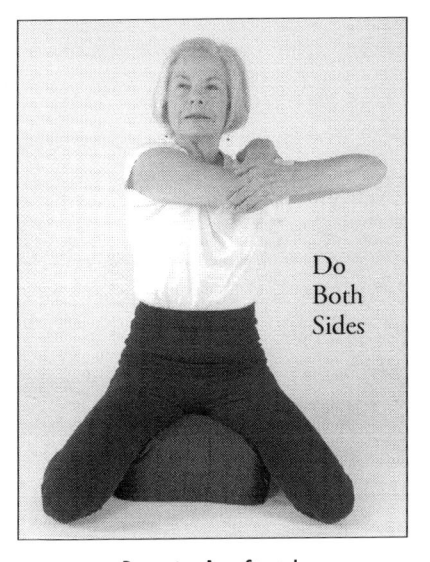

Posterior Arm Stretch

Also Stimulates the Following:

Three Leg Yin
Three Leg Yang

Three Arm Yin and Three Arm Yang *continued*

Also Stimulates the Following:

Anterior Thorax A
Three Leg Yin
Three Leg Yang

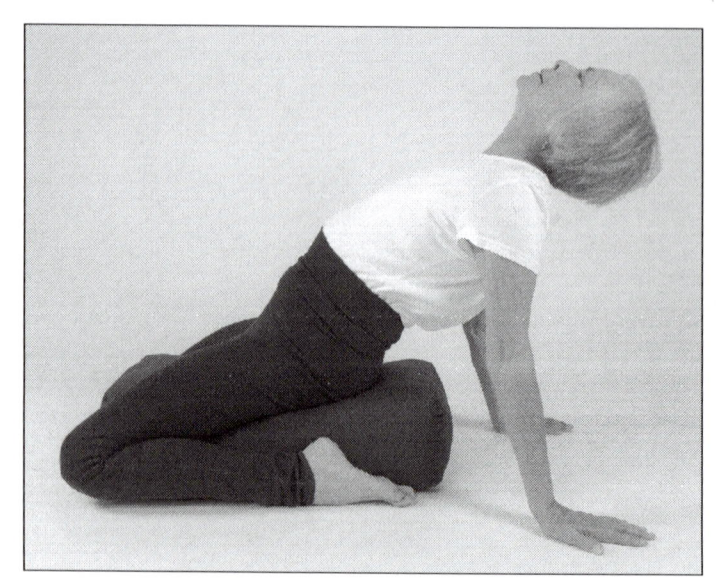

Ardha Supta Virasana with Palms Facing Out — Half Reclining Hero Pose

Also Stimulates the Following:

Anterior Thorax A
Three Leg Yin
Three Leg Yang

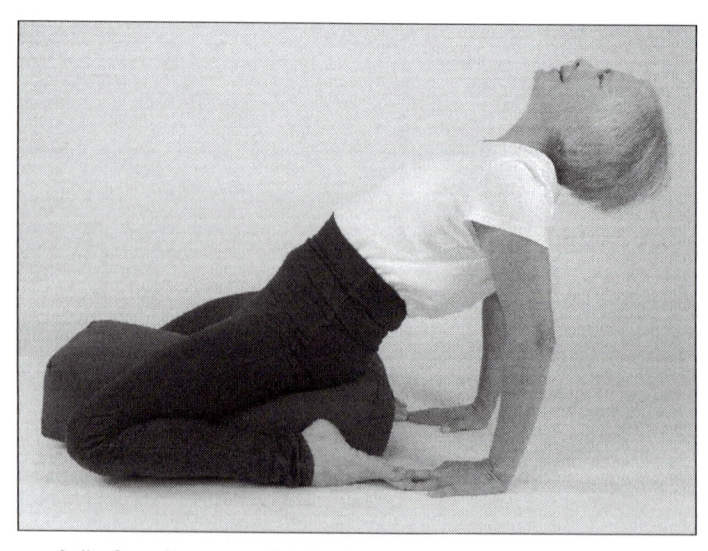

Ardha Supta Virasana with Palms Facing In — Half Reclining Hero Pose

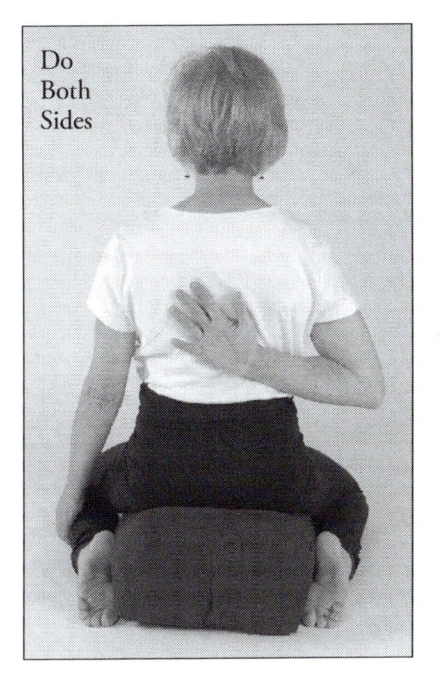

Three Arm Yin and Three Arm Yang 71

One Arm Gomukhasana —
One Arm Cow Face Pose

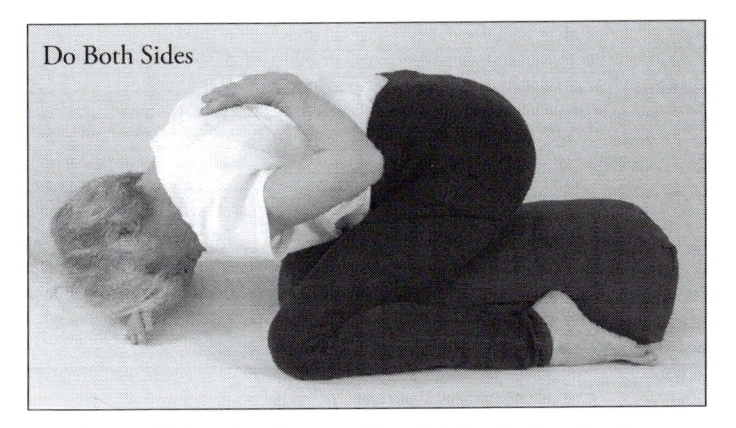

Also Stimulates the Following:

**Three Leg Yin
Three Leg Yang**

One Arm Utthita Gomukhasana — Extended One Arm Cow Face Pose

Also Stimulates the Following:

**Three Leg Yin
Three Leg Yang
Posterior Thorax**

Three Arm Yin and Three Arm Yang *continued*

Also Stimulates the Following:

Three Leg Yin

Three Leg Yang

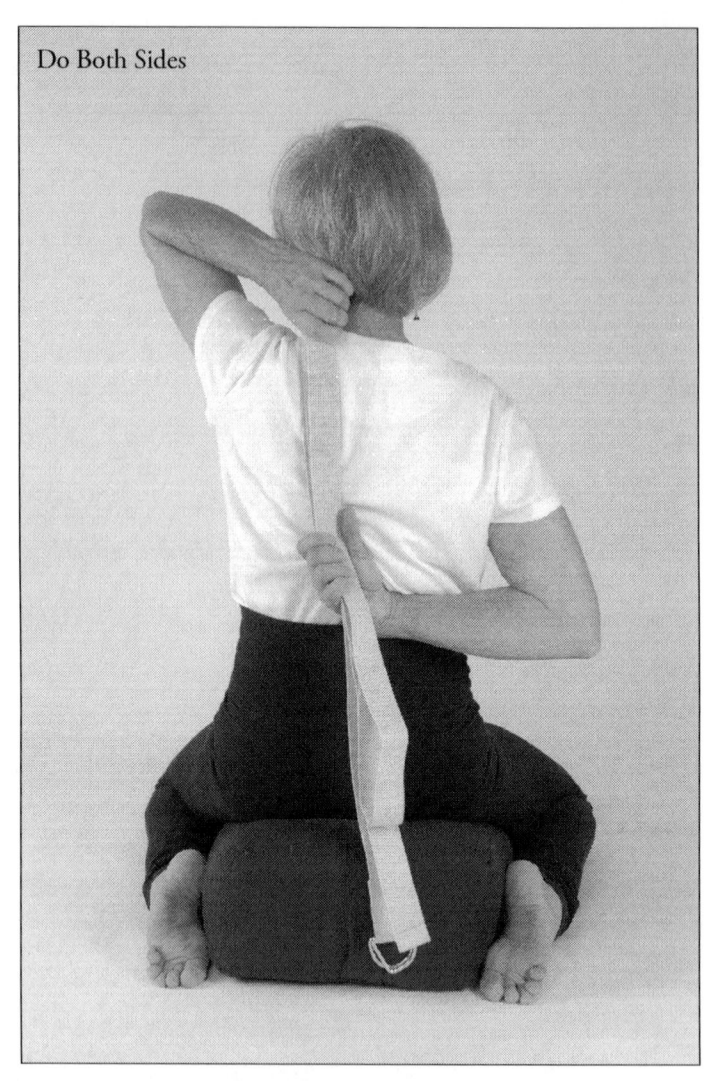

Do Both Sides

Gomukhasana Arms — Cow Face Pose Arms

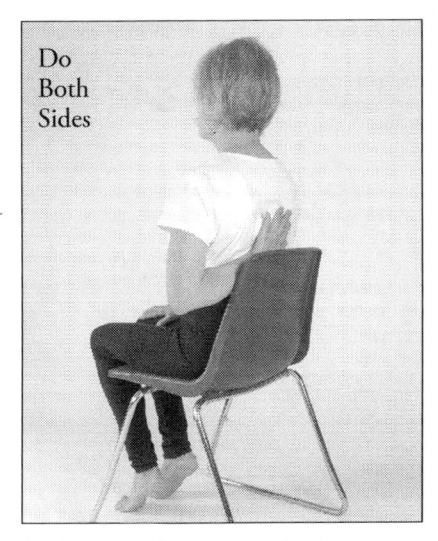

One Arm Gomukhasana with Palm Facing Out —
One Arm Cow Face Pose

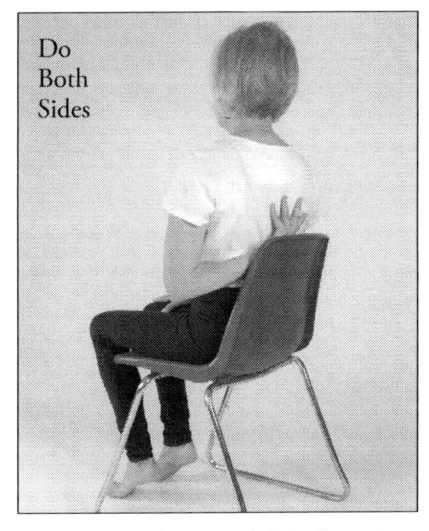

One Arm Gomukhasana with Palm Facing In —
One Arm Cow Face Pose

74 Meridian Systems Yoga

Three Arm Yin and Three Arm Yang *continued*

Also Stimulates the Following:

Three Leg Yin
Three Leg Yang

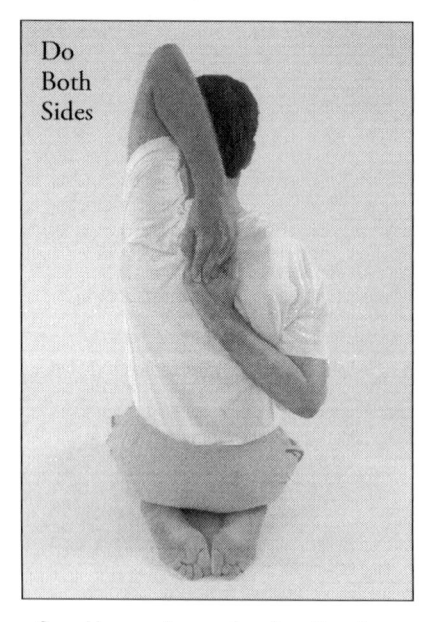

Do Both Sides

Gomukhasana Arms — Cow Face Pose Arms

Also Stimulates the Following:

Three Leg Yin
Three Leg Yang
Posterior Thorax

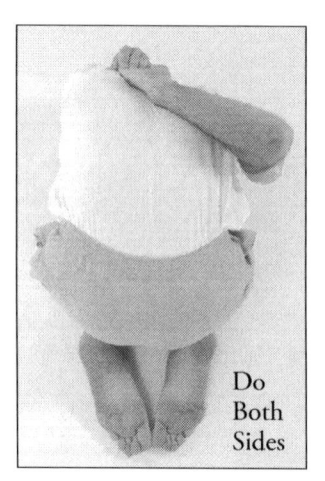

Do Both Sides

Utthita Gomukhasana Arms I —
Extended Cow Face Pose

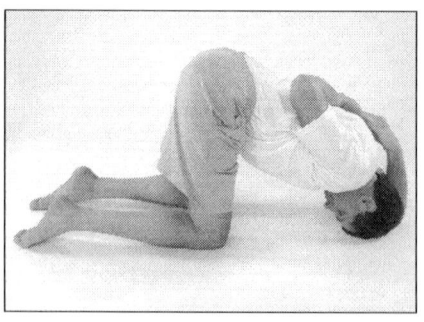

Utthita Gomukhasana Arms II —
Extended Cow Face Pose Arms

Three Arm Yin and Three Arm Yang 75

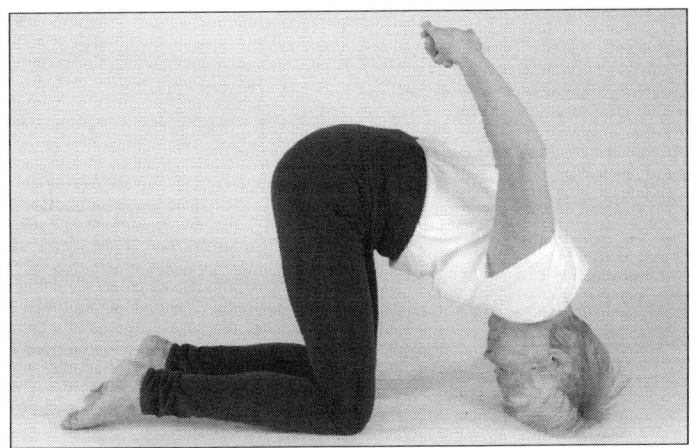

Utthita Gomukhasana Arms III - Extended Half Cow Face Pose

Also Stimulates the Following:

Posterior Thorax

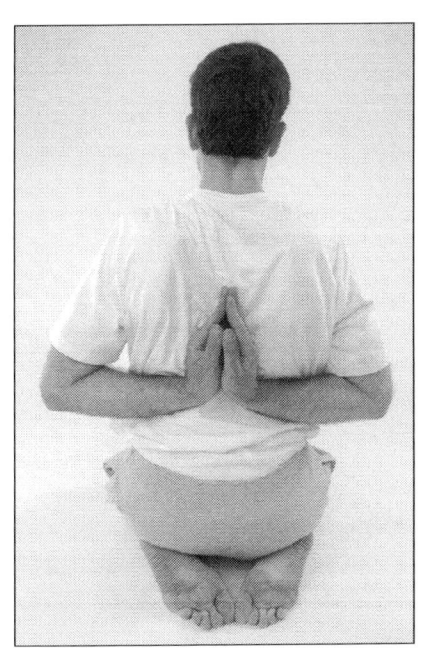

Viparita Namaskar — Inverted /Reverse Prayer

Also Stimulates the Following:

Three Leg Yin
Three Leg Yang

76 Meridian Systems Yoga

THREE LEG YIN AND THREE LEG YANG

Spleen and Stomach, Liver and Gall Bladder, Kidney and Urinary Bladder

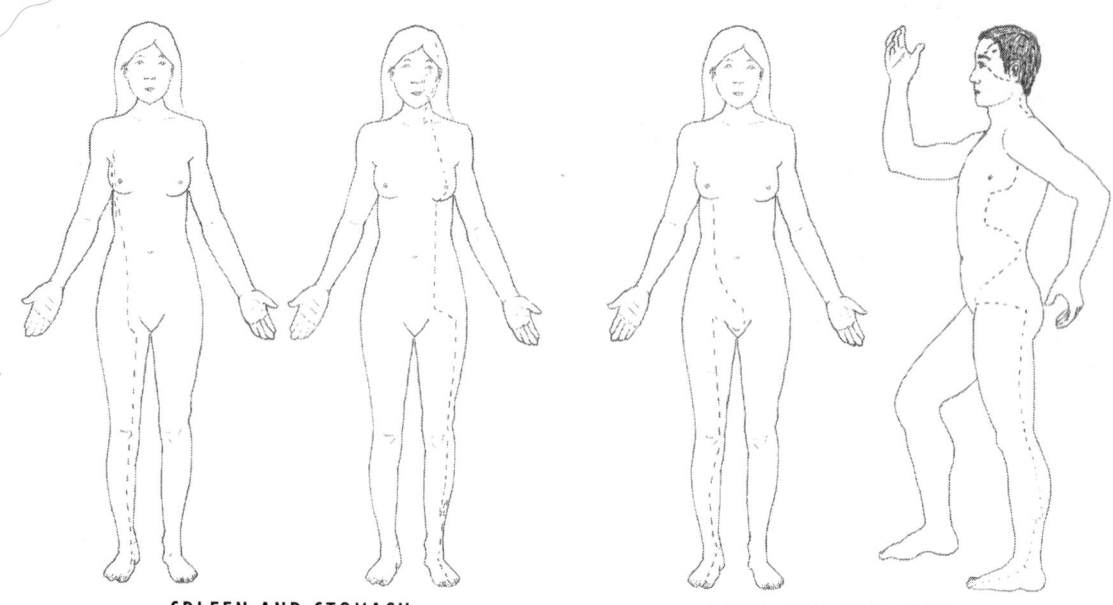

SPLEEN AND STOMACH

LIVER AND GALLBLADDER

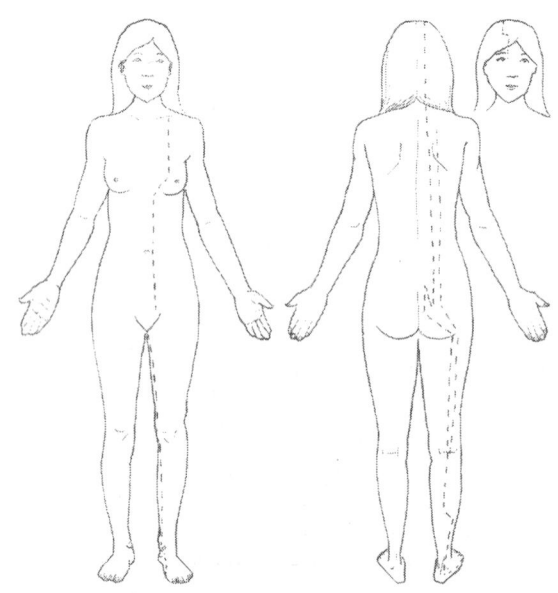

KIDNEY AND URINARY BLADDER

Three Leg Yin and Three Leg Yang

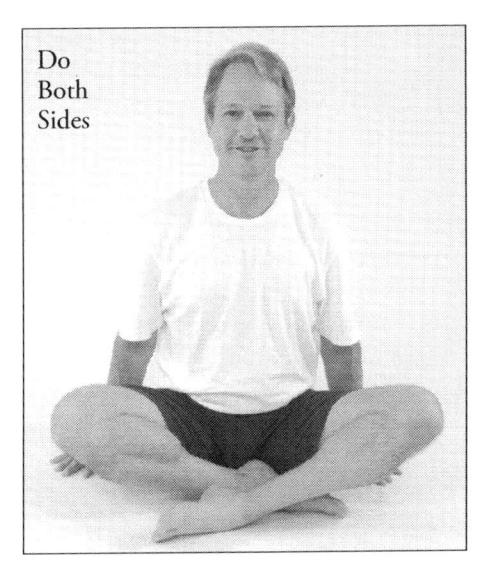

Do Both Sides

Sukhasana — Easy Pose

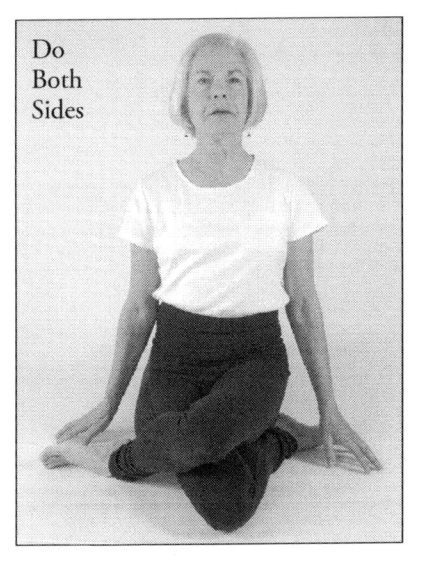

Do Both Sides

Gomukhaasana Legs — Cow Face Pose Legs

Three Leg Yin and Three Leg Yang *continued*

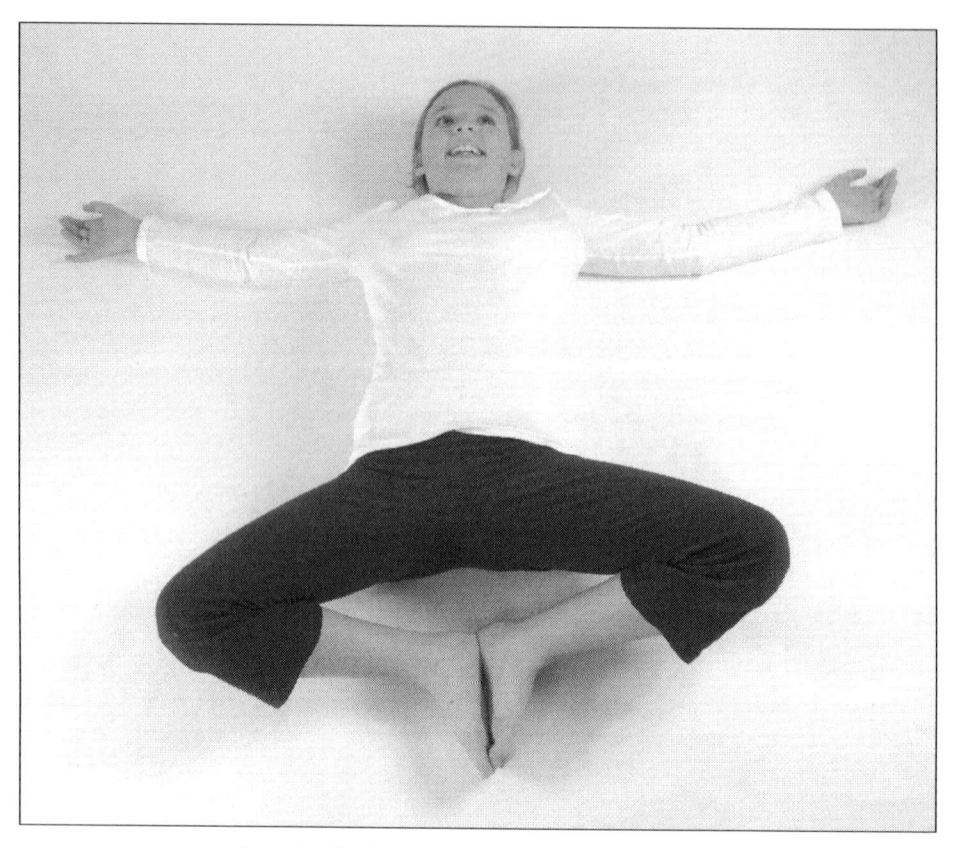

Supta Baddha Konasana — Reclining Bound Angle Pose

Three Leg Yin and Three Leg Yang 79

Do Both Sides

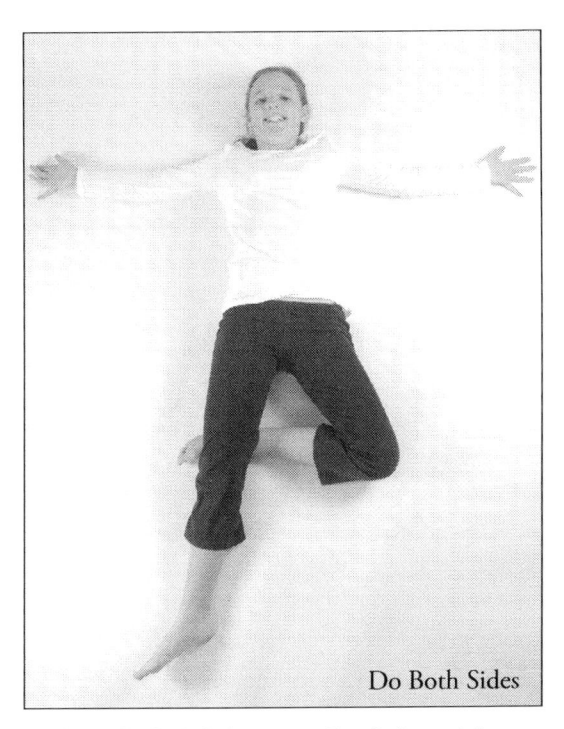

Supta Eka Pada Padmasana — Foot Underneath Leg
Reclining One Legged Lotus Pose

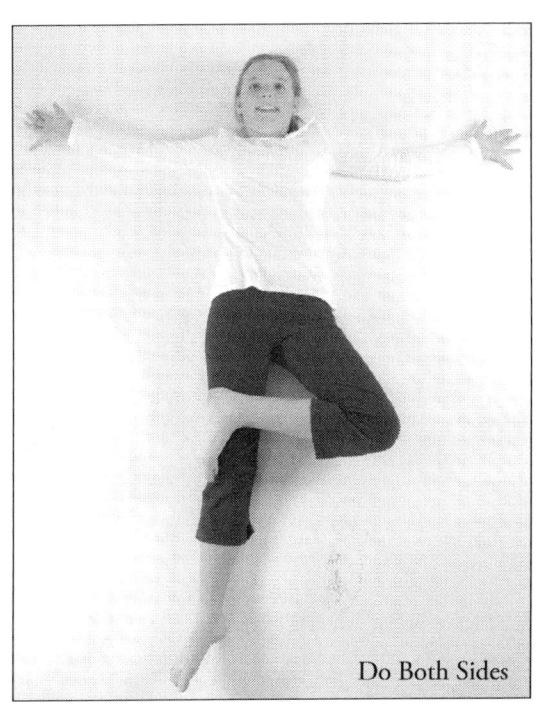

Do Both Sides

Supta Eka Pada Padmasana — Foot On Top of Leg
Reclining One Legged Lotus Pose

80 Meridian Systems Yoga

Three Leg Yin and Three Leg Yang *continued*

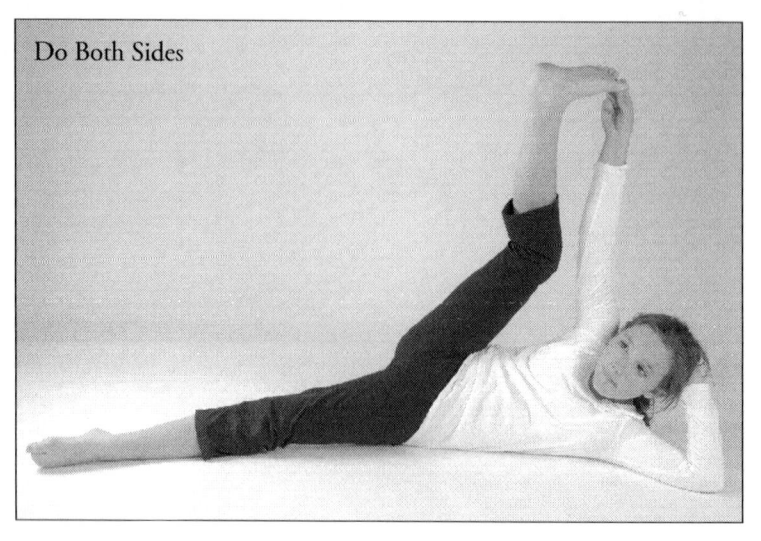

Do Both Sides

Anantasana — Sleeping Vishnu Pose

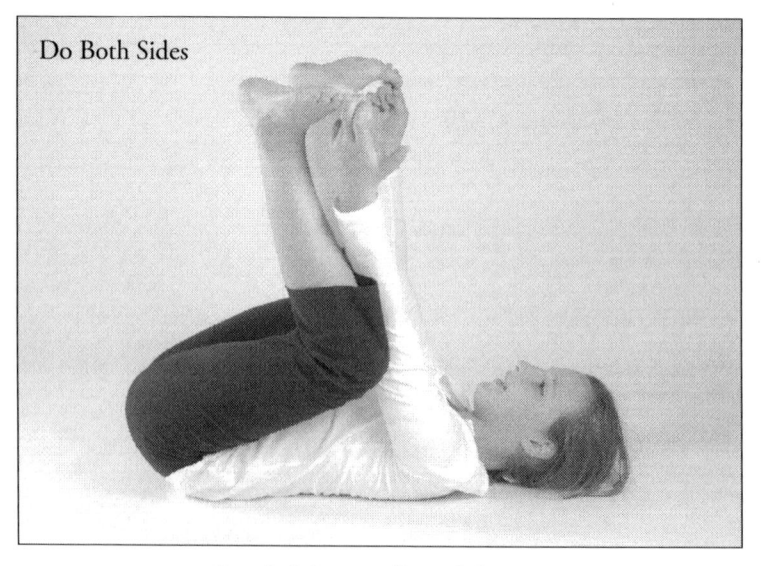

Do Both Sides

Ananda Balasana — Happy Baby Pose

Three Leg Yin and Three Leg Yang 81

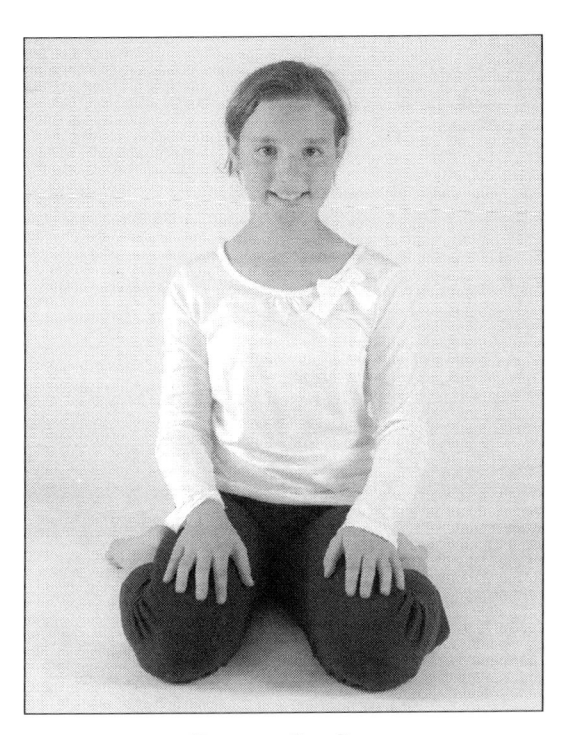

Virasana — Hero Pose

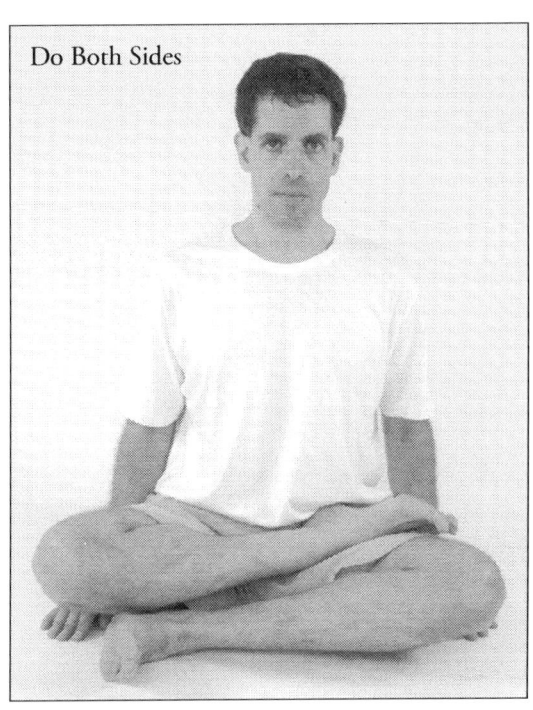

Do Both Sides

Eka Pada Padmasana — One Legged Lotus Pose

Meridian Systems Yoga Asana Sequences

Several asanas in the following asana sequence chapters may not fit the ability levels of all readers. Challenging asanas could be substituted with different asanas of the same meridian group. If you do not feel comfortable with any one of the asanas, stop and practice different asanas instead. The practice of this yoga method should always remain comfortable.

CHAPTER 12

Meridian Systems Yoga Asana Sequences

ANTERIOR & LATERAL THORAX, THREE LEG YIN & THREE LEG YANG

Spleen and Stomach, Liver and Gallbladder
  Nurture and Balance

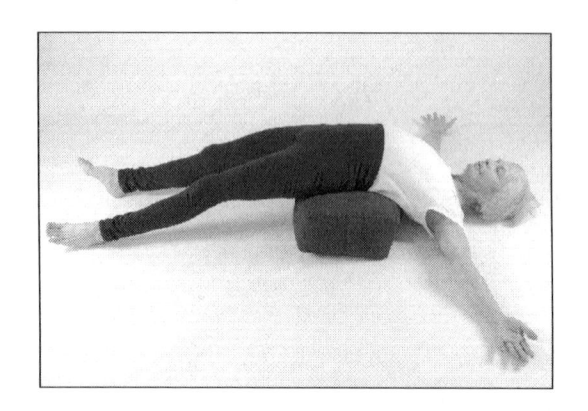

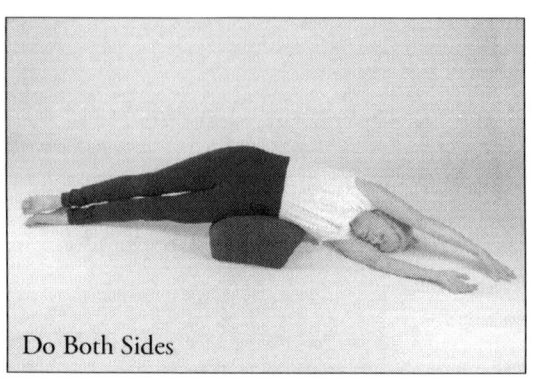

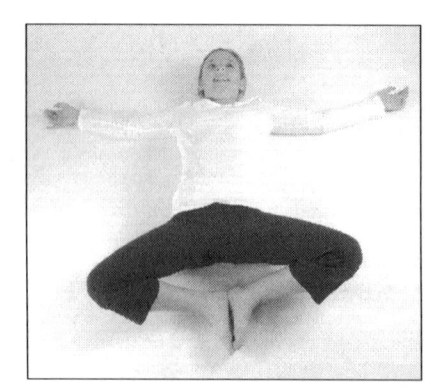

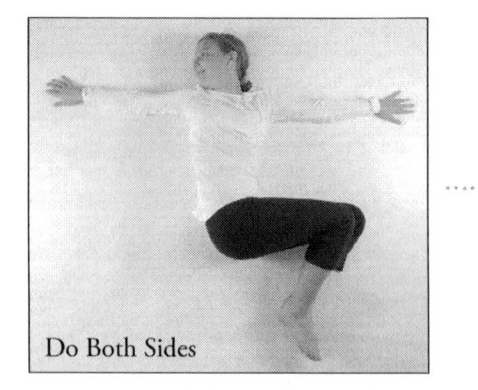

Do Both Sides

Do Both Sides

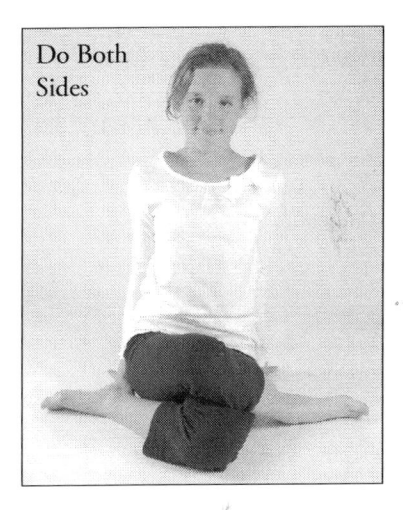

Anterior & Lateral Thorax, Three Leg Yin & Three Leg Yang

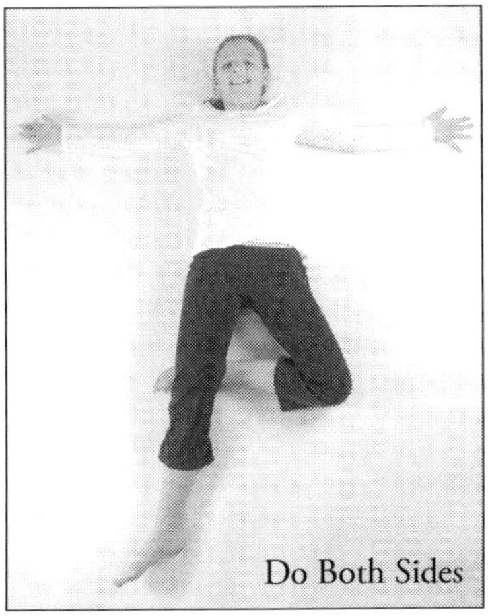

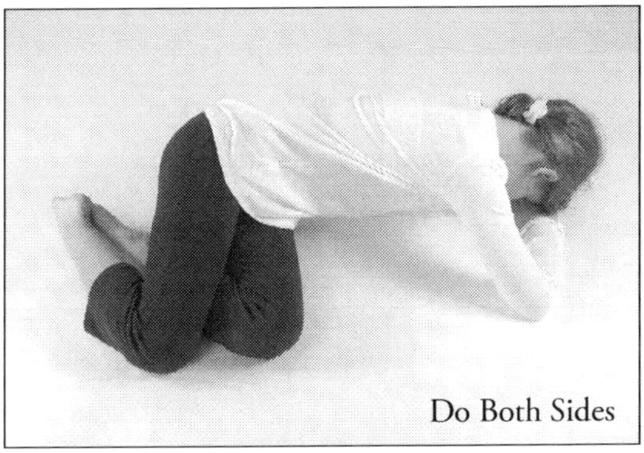

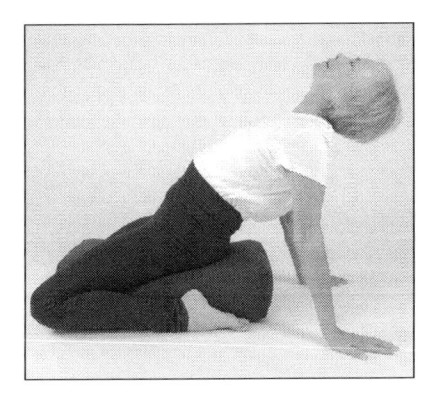

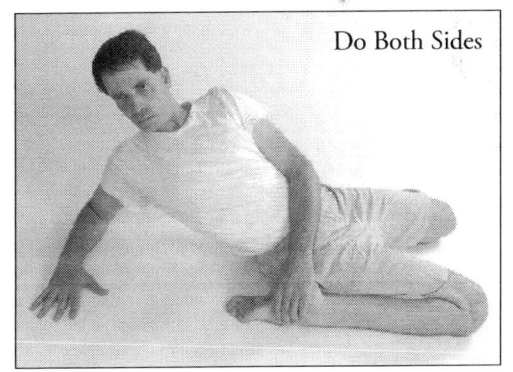

Do Both Sides

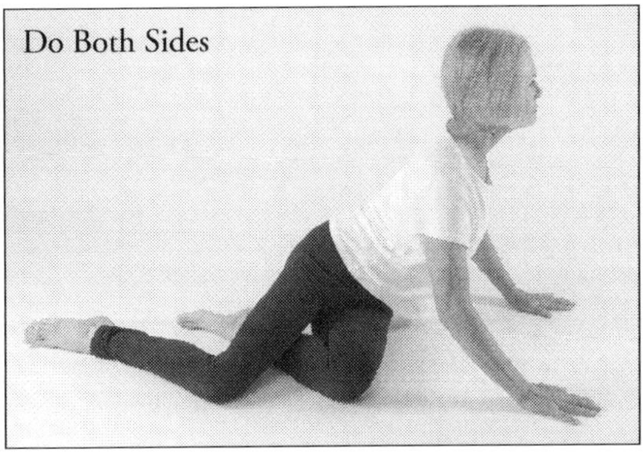

Do Both Sides

Do Both Sides

Do Both Sides

Do Both Sides

Do Both Sides

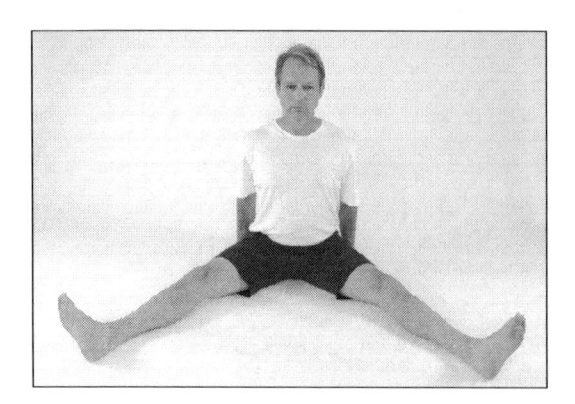

Anterior & Lateral Thorax, Three Leg Yin & Three Leg Yang *continued*

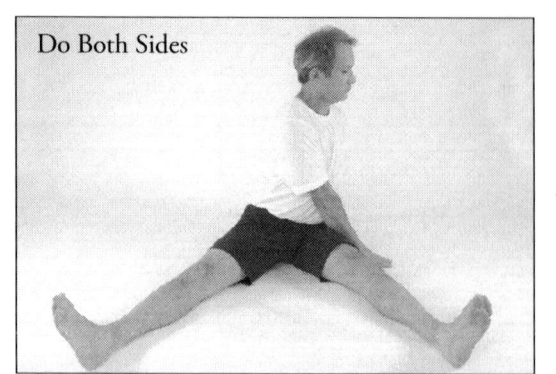

Do Both Sides

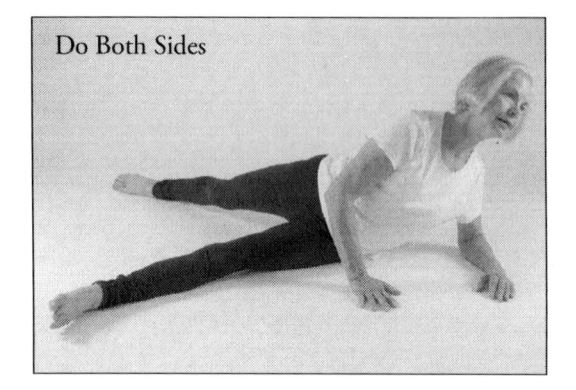

Do Both Sides

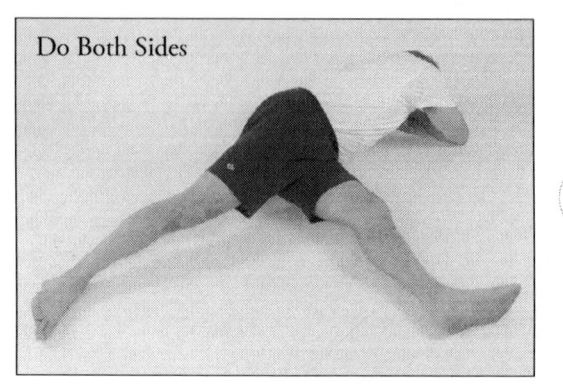

Do Both Sides

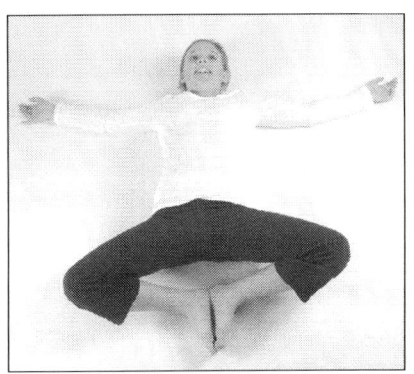

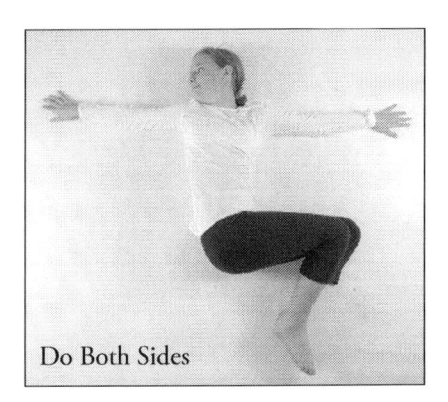

ANTERIOR & POSTERIOR THORAX, THREE LEG YIN & THREE LEG YANG
Sequence 1

Kidney and Urinary Bladder, Conception and Governing Vessel
  Strength and Truth

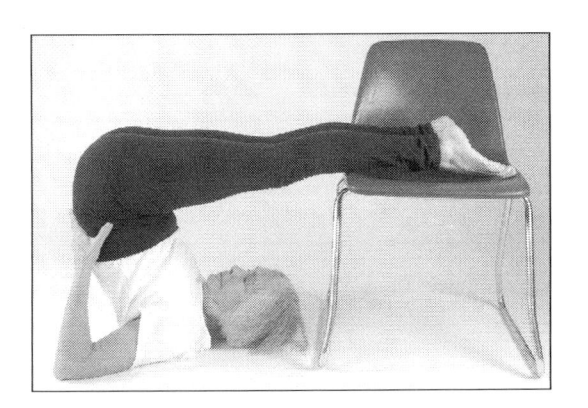

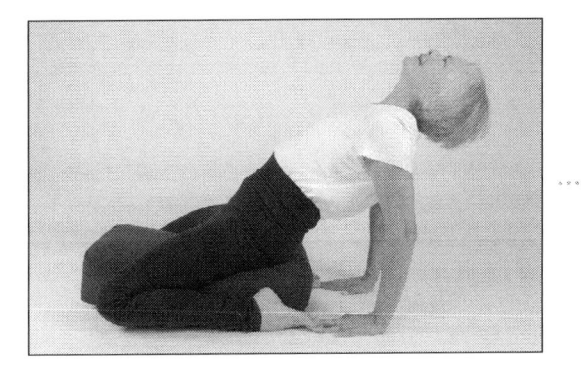

Do Both Sides

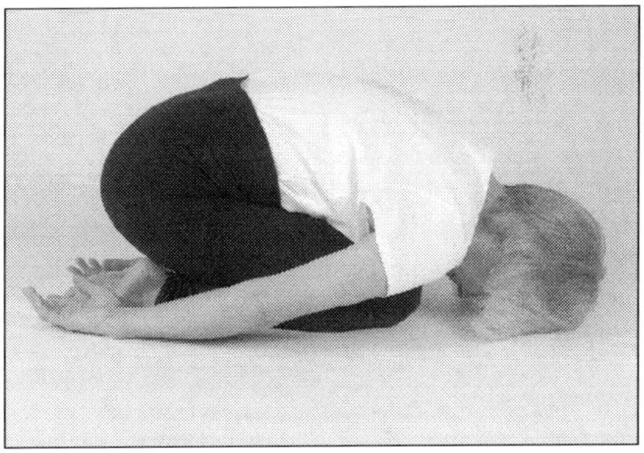

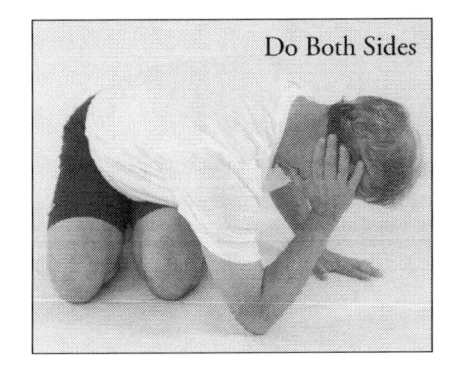

Do Both Sides

88 Meridian Systems Yoga

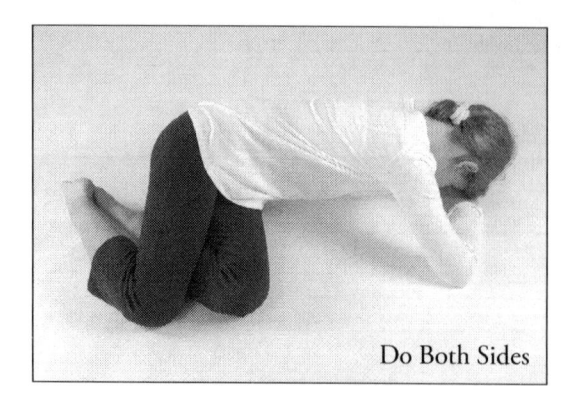

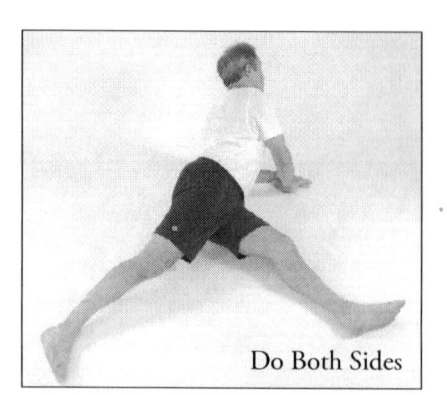

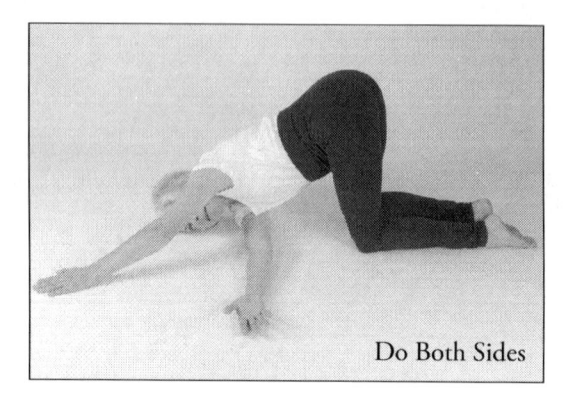

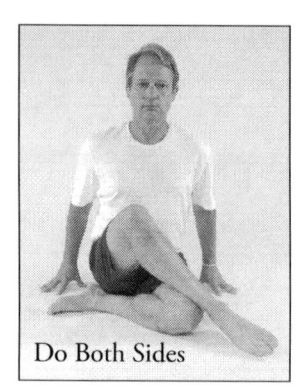

Anterior & Posterior Thorax, Three Leg Yin & Three Leg Yang *continued*

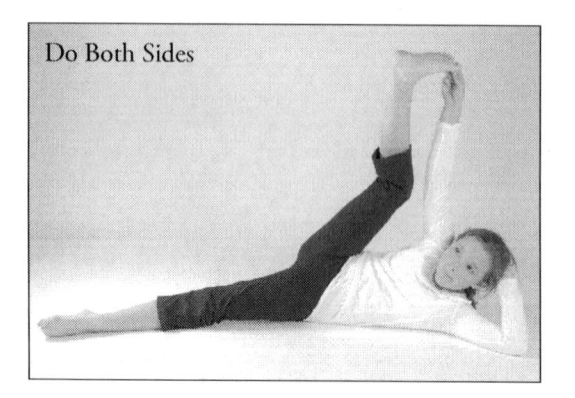

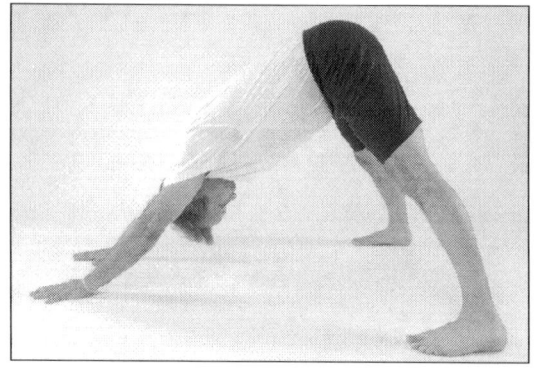

Do Both Sides

Do Both Sides

Do Both Sides

Do Both Sides

Do Both Sides

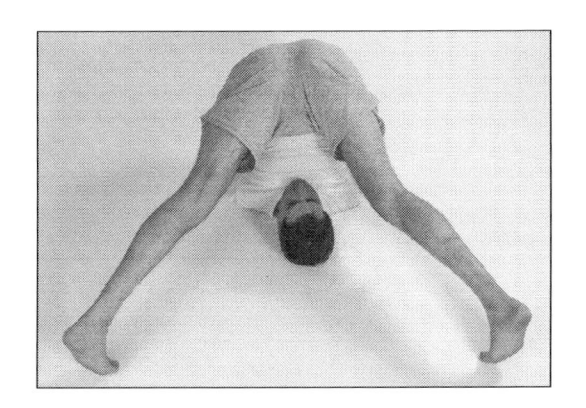

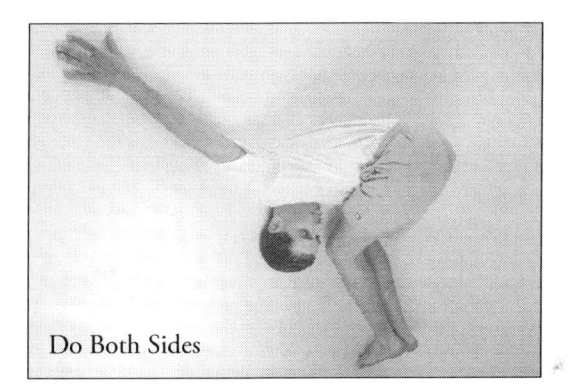

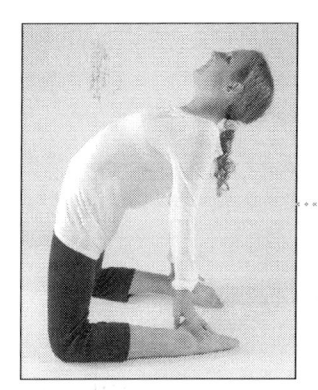

ANTERIOR & POSTERIOR THORAX, THREE LEG YIN & THREE LEG YANG
Sequence 2

Kidney and Urinary Bladder, Governing and Conception Vessels

Strength and Truth

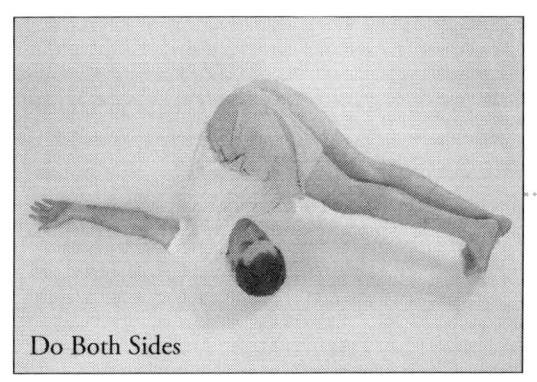

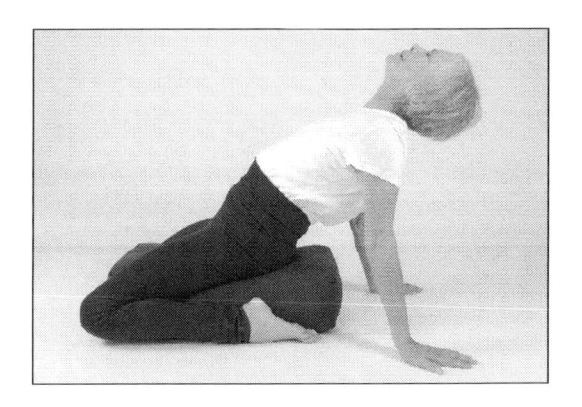

Do Both Sides

Do Both Sides

Do Both Sides

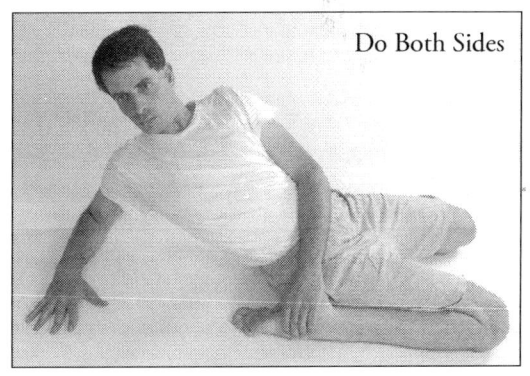

Do Both Sides

90 Meridian Systems Yoga

Anterior & Posterior Thorax, Three Leg Yin & Three Leg Yang *continued*

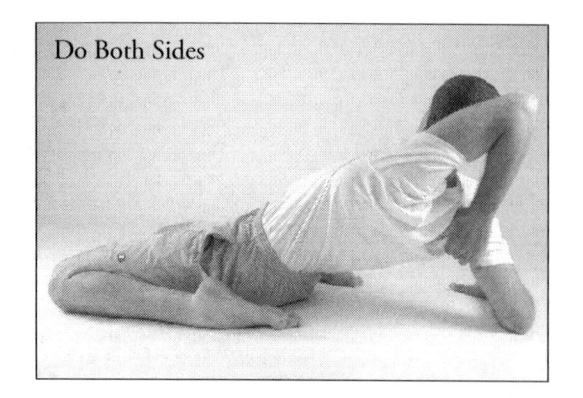

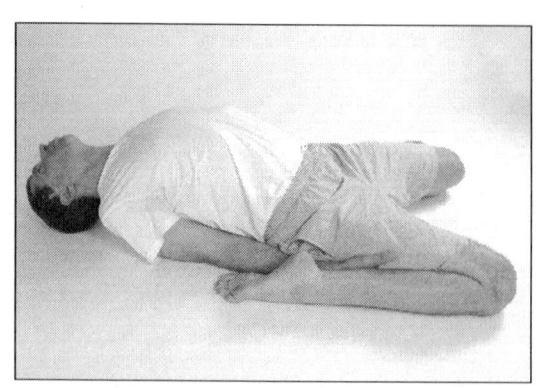

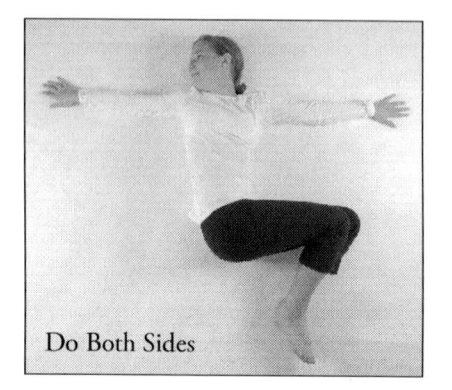

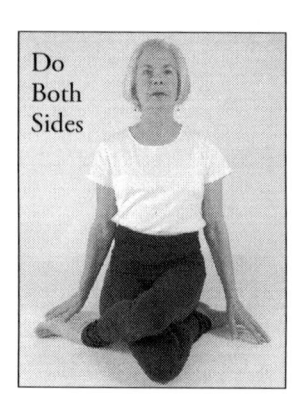

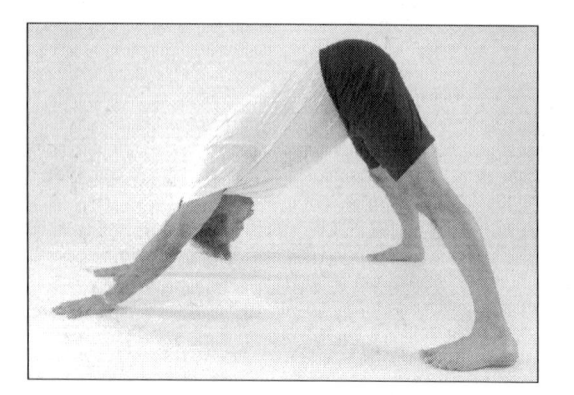

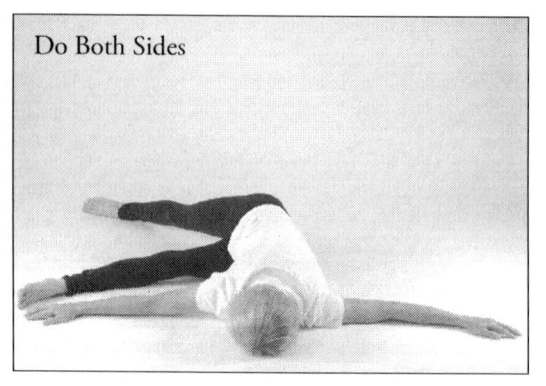

Do Both Sides

Do Both Sides

Do Both Sides

Do Both Sides

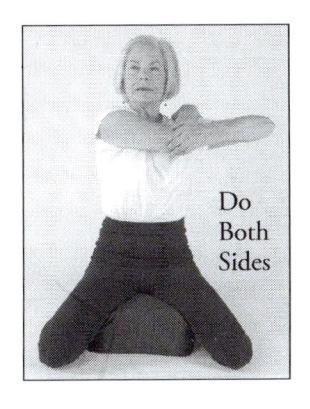

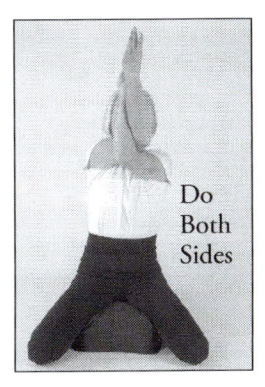

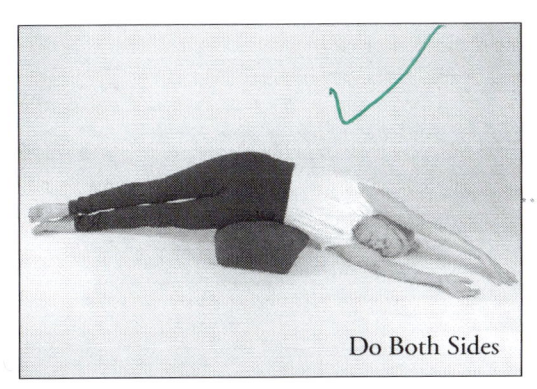

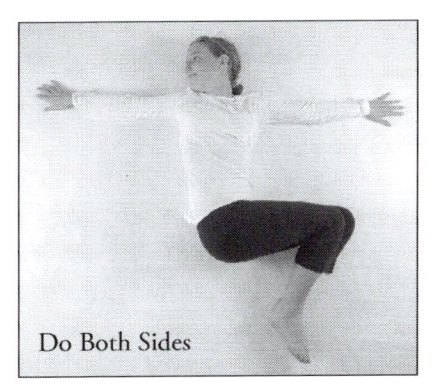

THREE ARM YIN & THREE ARM YANG

Lungs & Large Intestines, Heart & Small Intestines, Peridardium & Triple Burner
Integrity, Acceptance, Harmony

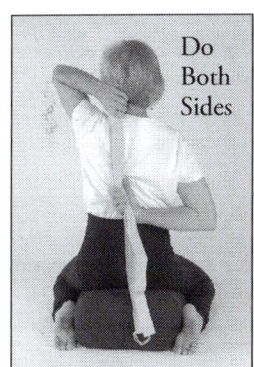

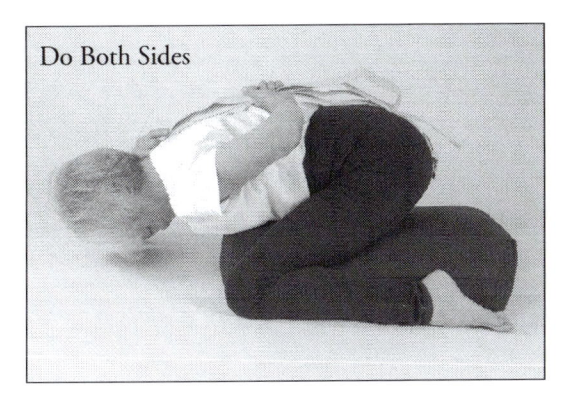

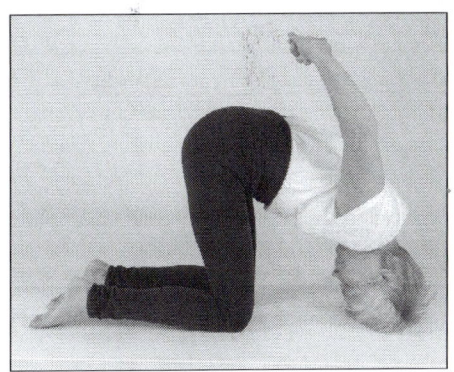

Do Both Sides

Do Both Sides

Do Both Sides

Do Both Sides

Do Both Sides

Do Both Sides

92 Meridian Systems Yoga

Three Arm Yin & Three Arm Yang *continued*

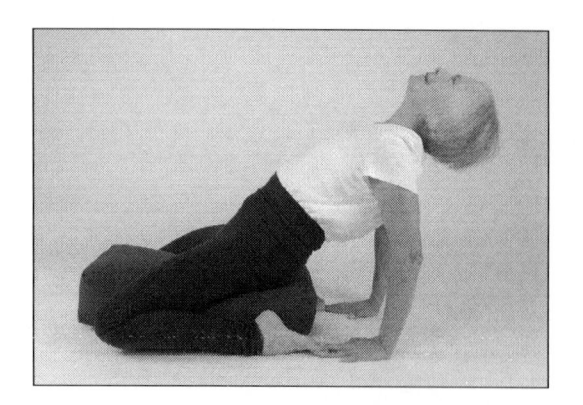

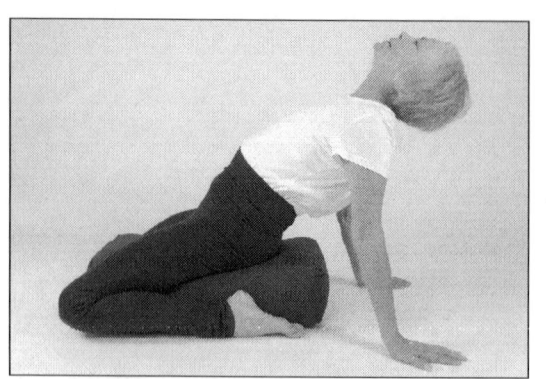

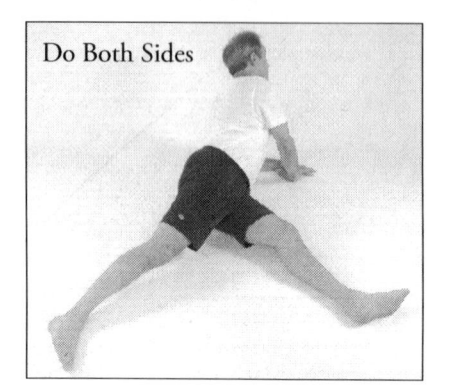

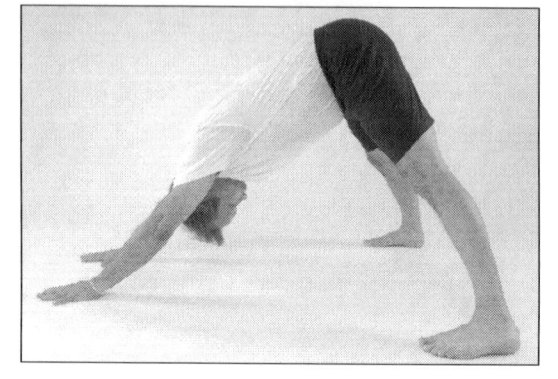

Do Both Sides

ALL MERIDIAN GROUPS ASANA SEQUENCE

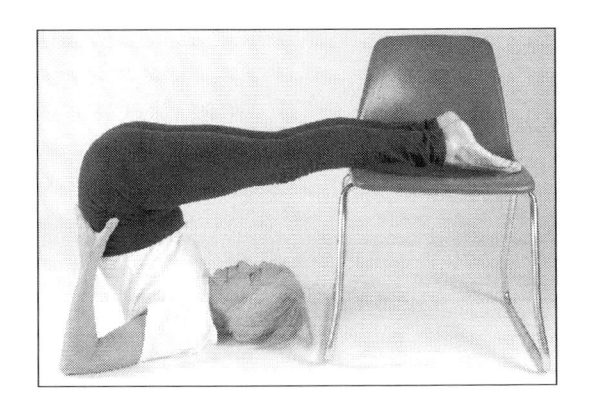

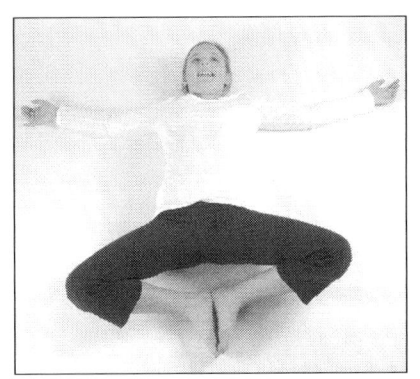

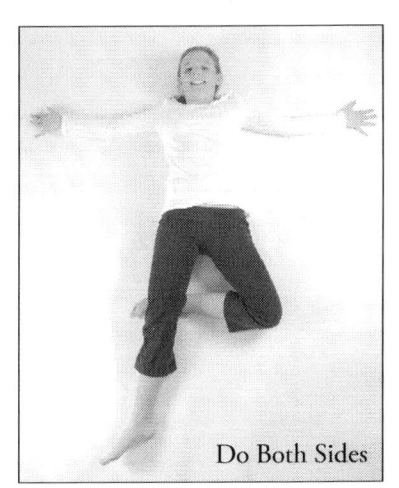

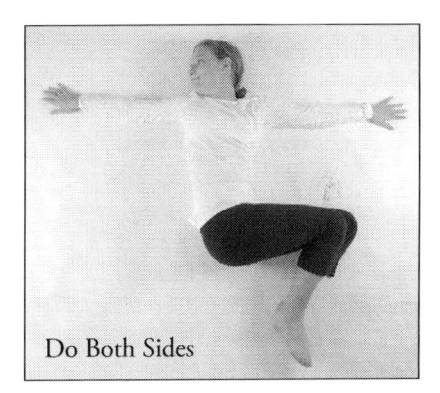

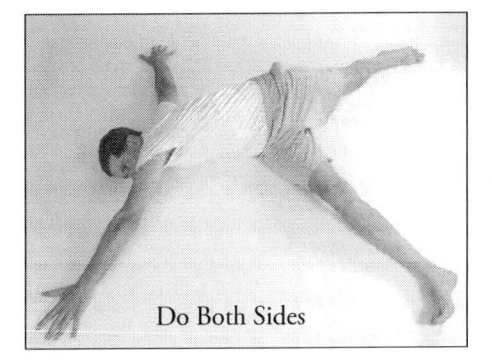

Do Both Sides

Do Both Sides

Do Both Sides

94　Meridian Systems Yoga

All Meridian Asana Groups Sequence *continued*

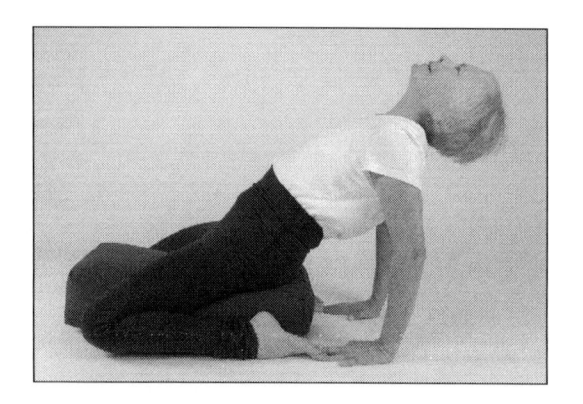

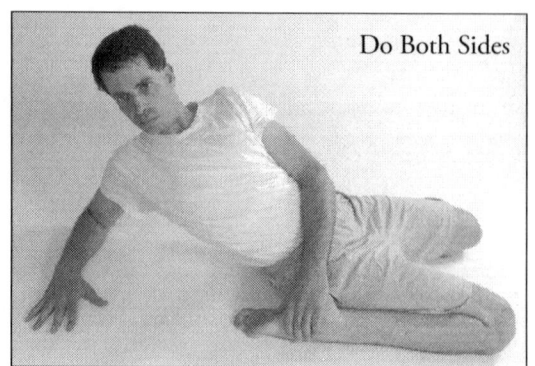

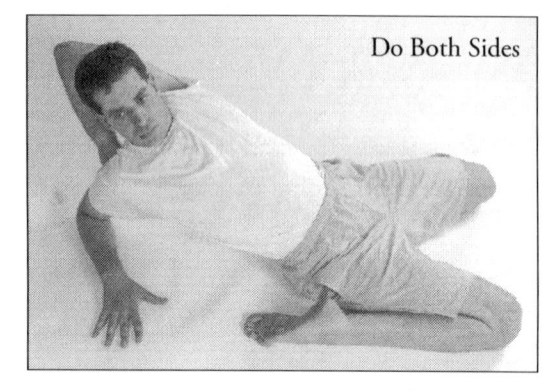

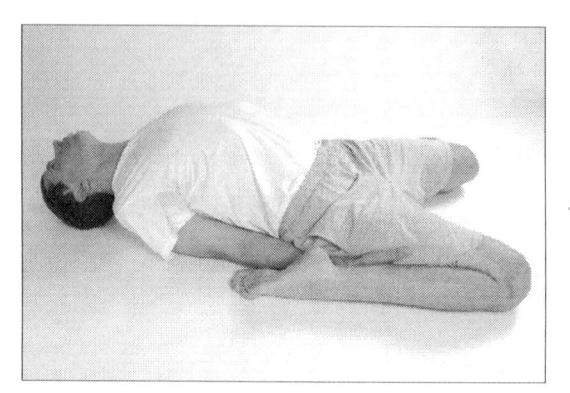

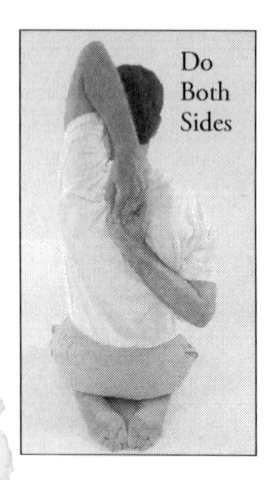

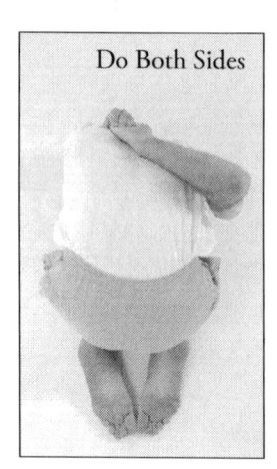

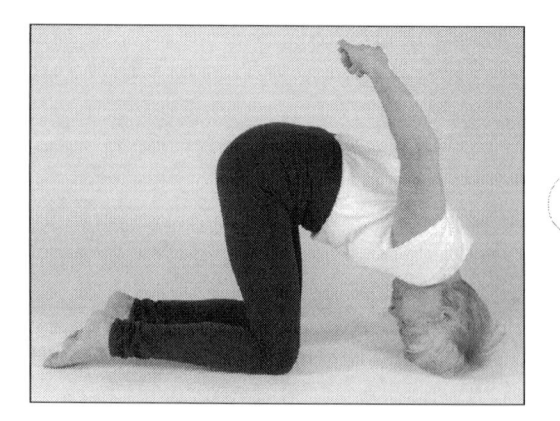

Do Both Sides

Do Both Sides

Do Both Sides

Do Both Sides

Do Both Sides

Bibliography and Suggested Reading

Acupuncture & Chinese Medicine

Deadman, Peter. *A Manual of Acupuncture.* East Sussex: Journal of Chinese Medicine Publications, 2011. Written by the chief editor of The Journal of Chinese Medicine, this book is a reference book of acupuncture points and channels.

Kapchuk, Ted. *The Web That Has No Weaver.* New York: McGraw-Hill, 2000. This book provides a rich introduction to Chinese medicine and is written in language that is suitable for the common reader.

Maciocia, Giovanni. *The Foundations of Chinese Medicine.* Philadelphia: Elsevier, 2005. This is a Chinese medicine textbook that gives an in-depth understanding of the theory of traditional Chinese medicine and acupuncture, with detailed use of acupuncture points and principles of treatment.

Ting, Esther and Marianne Jas. *Total Health the Chinese Way.* Philadelphia: Da Capo Press, 2009. This is a comprehensive guidebook for achieving overall health using TCM. The book includes a variety of exercises, tips, and dietary suggestions.

Yoga

Iyengar, B.K.S, *Light on Yoga.* New York: schocken Books, 1966 This book that has become a bible of yoga, written by one of the world's most famous yoga teachers.

Iyengar, B.K.S, *The Tree Of Yoga.* London: Aquarian Press, 1988. Another excellent review of yoga; its principals, philosophy, and practice.

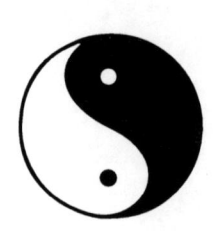

Printed in Great Britain
by Amazon.co.uk, Ltd.,
Marston Gate.